Infectious Diseases and Microbiology

New York

Infectious Diseases and Microbiology

Diseases Transmitted by Ticks
Hacer İşler (Editor)
Metin Özdemir, MD (Editor)
2021. ISBN: 978-1-68507-359-6 (Hardcover)
2021. ISBN: 978-1-68507-383-1 (eBook)

Impacts and Implications of COVID-19: An Analytical and Empirical Study
Anand Sharma (Editor)
Prateek Agrawal (Editor)
Vishu Madaan (Editor)
Anuj Agarwal (Editor)
2021. ISBN: 978-1-53619-670-2 (Hardcover)
2021. ISBN: 978-1-68507-081-6 (eBook)

Understanding the Spread of Infectious Diseases
Andrew J. Hinerman (Editor)
2020. ISBN: 978-1-53618-892-9 (Hardcover)
2020. ISBN: 978-1-53618-917-9 (eBook)

COVID-19 Pandemic: Questions, Answers and Hypotheses
A.K. Haghi (Editor)
2020. ISBN: 978-1-53618-565-2 (Softcover)
2020. ISBN: 978-1-53618-593-5 (eBook)

COVID 19
Sujith Ovallath, MBBS, MD, DNB, DM
2020. ISBN: 978-1-53618-691-8 (Softcover)
2020. ISBN: 978-1-53618-729-8 (eBook)

More information about this series can be found at
https://novapublishers.com/product-category/series/infectious-diseases-and-microbiology-new-in-2020/

Stefan Schneider
Editor

The Aviation Industry and COVID-19

snova
New York

Library of Congress Cataloging-in-Publication Data

ISBN: 978-1-68507-712-9

Published by Nova Science Publishers, Inc. † New York

Contents

Preface

International flight restrictions, local stay-at-home orders, and a general fear of contracting and spreading COVID-19 through air travel had a sudden and profound effect on the U.S. aviation industry. According to Department of Transportation (DOT) statistics, passenger traffic in April 2020 was 96 percent lower system-wide than April 2019, and remained 60 percent below 2019

This book examines the immediate effects of the COVID-19 pandemic on businesses across the aviation industry; actions those businesses took in response; actions the FAA took to help the industry respond to the pandemic; and the outlook for industry recovery, among other issues.

Chapter 1 - International flight restrictions, local stay-at-home orders, and a general fear of contracting and spreading COVID-19 through air travel had a sudden and profound effect on the U.S. aviation industry. According to Department of Transportation (DOT) statistics, passenger traffic in April 2020 was 96 percent lower system- wide than April 2019, and remained 60 percent below 2019 traffic levels throughout 2020.

This report examines (1) immediate effects of the COVID-19 pandemic on businesses across the aviation industry; (2) actions those businesses took in response; (3) actions the FAA took to help the industry respond to the pandemic; and (4) the outlook for industry recovery, among other issues.

GAO reviewed DOT airline operational and financial data from calendar years 2019 through 2020, financial statements from various aviation- related businesses, FAA regulations and operational guidance, and industry recovery forecasts. GAO conducted a generalizable survey of 1,136 smaller airports. GAO also interviewed officials from FAA and representatives from a judgmental sample of 47 aviation and aerospace industry stakeholders selected based on location and industry sector.

Chapter 2 - Within TSA, approximately 46,000 TSOs stationed across the nation's commercial airports perform screening and other activities that often require close interaction with passengers. As a result, both passengers and

TSOs may be at an increased risk of infection during pandemics such as COVID-19.

The CARES Act included a provision for GAO to conduct monitoring and oversight of the federal government's response to the COVID-19 pandemic. This report identifies 1) what steps TSA has taken to reduce the spread of COVID-19 at passenger screening checkpoints; and 2) how TSA is monitoring TSOs' implementation of amended safety and screening procedures, among other objectives.

GAO analyzed TSA data on TSOs' use of paid leave, reviewed documentation on policies and procedures, and interviewed TSA officials at headquarters and eight U.S. airports. We selected these airports to reflect diversity in the number of COVID-19 cases among TSOs, airport size, and geographic region. In addition, for six of these airports, GAO reviewed closed circuit television footage to observe how TSOs were implementing COVID-19 procedural changes.

Chapter 3 - In the U.S. there have been over 29 million cumulative reported cases of COVID-19 and about 524,000 reported deaths, as of March 23, 2021. Public health officials have recommended social distancing and other steps to reduce the spread of the disease, but air marshals often work on planes where they cannot fully adopt these measures. The CARES Act included a provision for GAO to conduct monitoring and oversight of the federal government's response to the COVID- 19 pandemic. This report examines (1) how many air marshals have been diagnosed with COVID-19; (2) FAMS's steps to protect air marshals' health; and (3) how FAMS adapted its operations during the pandemic.

GAO analyzed FAMS data on COVID- 19 cases among employees, reviewed agency guidance, analyzed FAMS flight operations reports, and interviewed FAMS leadership as well as air marshals at a non-generalizable sample of three field offices selected for variation in number of COVID-19 cases, among other things. This is a public version of a sensitive report that GAO issued in May 2021. Information that DHS deemed sensitive has been omitted.

Chapter 1

COVID-19 Pandemic: Observations on the Ongoing Recovery of the Aviation Industry*

United States Government Accountability Office

Why GAO Did This Study

International flight restrictions, local stay-at-home orders, and a general fear of contracting and spreading COVID-19 through air travel had a sudden and profound effect on the U.S. aviation industry. According to Department of Transportation (DOT) statistics, passenger traffic in April 2020 was 96 percent lower system- wide than April 2019, and remained 60 percent below 2019 traffic levels throughout 2020.

This report examines (1) immediate effects of the COVID-19 pandemic on businesses across the aviation industry; (2) actions those businesses took in response; (3) actions the FAA took to help the industry respond to the pandemic; and (4) the outlook for industry recovery, among other issues.

GAO reviewed DOT airline operational and financial data from calendar years 2019 through 2020, financial statements from various aviation- related businesses, FAA regulations and operational guidance, and industry recovery forecasts. GAO conducted a generalizable survey of 1,136 smaller airports. GAO also interviewed officials from FAA and representatives from a judgmental sample of 47 aviation and aerospace industry stakeholders selected based on location and industry sector.

---

* This is an edited, reformatted and augmented version of United States Government Accountability Office, Publication No. GAO-22-104429, dated October 2021.

In: The Aviation Industry and COVID-19
Editor: Stefan Schneider
ISBN: 978-1-68507-712-9

What GAO Recommends

GAO continues to urge Congress to take legislative action to require DOT to work with relevant agencies, stakeholders, and members of the aviation and public health sectors to develop a national aviation- preparedness plan for communicable disease threats.

What GAO Found

The COVID-19 pandemic severely affected the aviation and aerospace sectors that depend on commercial passenger travel. As demand for air travel plummeted and remained low throughout 2020, effects cascaded across sectors including U.S. passenger airlines, airports, aviation manufacturers, and repair station operators. For example, in response to reduced demand, airlines parked or retired a substantial portion of their aircraft fleet, which, in turn, reduced demand for aircraft maintenance services.

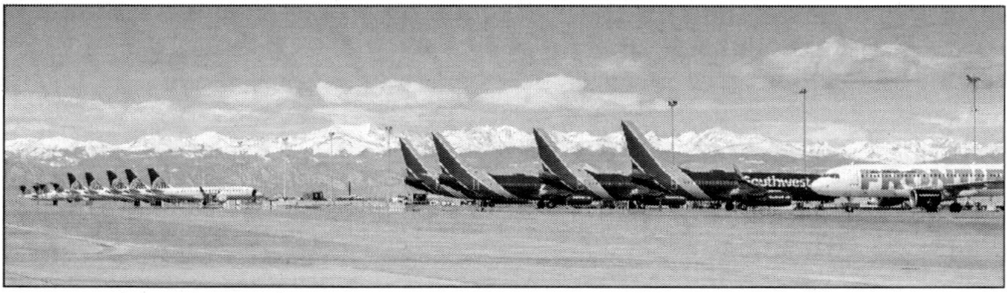

Source: Denver International Airport. | GAO-22-104429.

Aircraft Temporarily Stored at Denver International Airport in 2020.

In response to the pandemic's effects, aviation stakeholders reported that they acted quickly to mitigate financial losses and position themselves to maintain business viability until demand increased. Stakeholders' actions included:

- managing costs, such as by implementing early retirement programs;
- raising funds in the private market to increase liquidity; and
- taking steps to mitigate COVID-19's spread among employees and customers.

Stakeholders also noted the importance of the over $100 billion in payroll support payments, loans, and other financial assistance provided through COVID-19 relief legislation.

The Federal Aviation Administration (FAA) reported taking quick action to help the aviation industry adjust operations in response to the pandemic. These actions included providing temporary relief from some regulatory requirements— such as airline crewmember medical certifications—and issuing guidance to airlines and airports on mitigating COVID-19 risks. FAA has phased out many of these relief measures.

Although airlines experienced a rebound in demand for U.S. leisure travel in 2021, operational challenges and concerns about the COVID-19 Delta variant have slowed recovery. Forecasts suggest that industry recovery will be uneven as business and international air travel—the most profitable segments—are likely to lag. Stakeholders identified areas of concern for policymakers to consider, such as strengthening aviation workforce pipelines, as they determine how or whether to continue to assist the industry in evolving market conditions. Further, developing a national aviation-preparedness plan for communicable disease, as GAO recommended, would provide greater coordination among federal and industry stakeholders and help better prepare the U.S. for future pandemics.

Abbreviations

A4A	Airlines for America
AMTS	Aviation Maintenance Technician School
ARC	Airlines Reporting Corporation
ARSA	Aeronautical Repair Station Association
BLS	Bureau of Labor Statistics
BTS	Bureau of Transportation Statistics
CARES	Coronavirus Aid, Relief, and Economic Security
CDC	Centers for Disease Control and Prevention
COVID-19	Coronavirus Disease 2019
DHS	Department of Homeland Security
DOT	Department of Transportation
EAS	Essential Air Service
FAA	Federal Aviation Administration
FBO	fixed base operator
HHS	Department of Health and Human Services

NPIAS	National Plan of Integrated Airport Systems
OEM	original equipment manufacturer
PFC	passenger facility charge
PPP	Paycheck Protection Program
PSP	Payroll Support Program
SCASDP	Small Community Air Service Development Program
SEC	Securities and Exchange Commission
SFAR	Special Federal Aviation Regulation
Treasury	Department of the Treasury
TSA	Transportation Security Administration
UAS	uncrewed aircraft systems

October 21, 2021
Congressional Addressees

The Coronavirus Disease 2019 (COVID-19) pandemic has resulted in catastrophic loss of life and substantial damage to the global economy. The global aviation industry was among those most severely affected. International flight restrictions, local stay-at-home orders, and a general fear of contracting and spreading COVID-19 through air travel had a sudden and profound effect on the global aviation industry, including passenger airlines, airports, and the entire ecosystem of businesses that supply, manufacture, and repair commercial and general aviation aircraft.

According to Bureau of Transportation Statistics (BTS) data, U.S. airline passenger traffic was down 60 percent system-wide in 2020 compared to 2019 traffic levels.[1] The ripple effect from this unprecedented and sustained reduction in demand throughout 2020 has affected airline business models, employment, and the entire aviation supply chain.[2] In response to the

[1] BTS is the Department of Transportation's source for commercial aviation, multimodal freight activity, and transportation economics.

[2] For example, according to the Bureau of Labor Statistics (BLS), as of April 2021—the most recent data available—an estimated 136,400 jobs in the air transportation and support activities sectors—approximately 22 percent—have been lost since peak employment levels of 755,400 in February 2020, although employment has risen roughly 7 percent since October 2020. According to BLS, the air transportation sector includes scheduled air carriers that fly regular routes on regular schedules and operate even if flights are only partially loaded, and non-scheduled carriers that provide chartered air transportation of passengers, cargo, or specialty flying services and often operate at nonpeak time slots at busy airports. Among other things, the support activities for air transportation sector includes airport operations and air traffic control.

pandemic, the Coronavirus Aid, Relief, and Economic Security (CARES) Act and subsequent COVID-19 relief laws appropriated over $100 billion to provide financial assistance to the U.S. aviation industry and its workers.[3]

You asked us to conduct a broad review to gather input from a wide range of stakeholders, including airlines, airports, aviation labor, general aviation users, commercial space companies and others, on several key issues related to the industry and federal response to the COVID-19 pandemic, including:

- the effects of the COVID-19 pandemic on selected aviation and aerospace industry sectors in 2020;
- actions selected aviation and aerospace stakeholders took in response to the pandemic;
- actions taken by the Federal Aviation Administration to help the aviation industry respond to the pandemic, and selected aviation stakeholders' perspectives on those actions; and
- the outlook for aviation industry recovery, and stakeholder considerations for potential federal support in assisting the aviation industry in the future.

To identify the effects of the pandemic on selected aviation industry sectors and their respective responses to the pandemic, we analyzed the Department of Transportation's (DOT) Form 41 financial and operational data for calendar years 2019 and 2020. We determined that these data were sufficiently reliable for the purposes of our reporting objectives by reviewing the quality control procedures used by DOT. We also analyzed financial statements reported to the Securities and Exchange Commission (SEC) by publicly-traded airlines and other aviation-related businesses from the first quarter through the fourth quarter of 2020 to obtain quantitative information on their financial performance, as well as qualitative descriptions of the impact of the pandemic on businesses and actions those businesses took in response.[4] We reported on the immediate effects of the pandemic based on the expectation that other effects will be long-term. We conducted interviews with a judgmental sample of 47 aviation and aerospace industry stakeholders—including passenger airlines, cargo airlines, large and medium hub airports, and aviation manufacturers—on the effects of the COVID-19 pandemic on

[3] CARES Act, Pub. L. No. 116-136, §§ 4003, 4112, 134 Stat. 281, 470, 498 (2020); Consolidated Appropriations Act, 2021, Pub. L. No. 116-260, div. N, tit. IV, 134 Stat. 1182, 2052-61 (2020); American Rescue Plan Act of 2021, Pub. L. No. 117-2, § 7301, 135 Stat. 4, 104-107.

[4] The four quarters cover the 12 months of calendar year 2020.

selected aviation and aerospace industry sectors and actions stakeholders took in response.[5]

We also conducted a generalizable, web-based survey of smaller airports— including small hub, non-hub, non-primary commercial service, general aviation, and reliever airports—to identify the effects of the pandemic on these airports and actions they took in response.[6] The survey response rate was 72 percent.[7] Estimates generated from these survey results are generalizable to the target population of 2,752 smaller airports in the continental U.S.[8]

To identify the actions the Federal Aviation Administration (FAA) took to help the aviation industry respond to the pandemic, we reviewed requests for regulatory relief submitted to FAA by aviation stakeholders and FAA's related rulemakings, exemptions, and extensions, as well as operational guidance. We interviewed officials from FAA divisions responsible for implementing these actions as well as those of the 47 aviation and aerospace stakeholders selected whose operations were potentially affected by these actions.

---

[5] We selected aviation and aerospace industry stakeholders to represent a cross-section of sectors within the aviation and aerospace industries as well as based on geographic representation. The stakeholders we selected include an analytics and engineering firm; 9 industry associations; 2 aviation labor organizations; 6 passenger airlines; 3 cargo airlines; 5 aviation manufacturers; 3 repair station operators; 11 large and medium hub airports; 2 commercial space launch providers; 3 credit rating agencies, and 2 aviation industry analysts.

[6] We conducted the survey from November 16 through December 11, 2020. We used a sampling frame of 2,752 airports (64 small hub, 209 non-hub, 63 non-primary commercial service, and 2,416 general aviation and reliever airports). Large and medium hub airports, non-primary airports with an unclassified role, airports outside of the continental U.S., and proposed airports were excluded from the sample frame. Small hub airports are those that account for at least 0.05 but less than 0.25 percent of annual passenger enplanements; non-hub airports are those that account for less than 0.05 percent of passenger enplanements but have more than 10,000 enplanements annually; non-primary commercial service airports have at least 2,500 and no more than 10,000 annual enplanements.

[7] This is the unweighted response rate. The weighted response rate was 65 percent. Following best practices in survey research and in Office of Management and Budget, *Standards and Guidelines for Statistical Surveys* (September 2006), we carried out a nonresponse bias analysis. The nonresponse bias analysis and subsequent weighted adjustments only included variables available on the National Plan of Integrated Airport Systems (NPIAS) sample frame and did not account for unobserved variables that could potentially be related to the likelihood of response. However, based on our knowledge of aviation operations, we did not expect survey responses or the likelihood of response to vary by other airport characteristics. Based on this nonresponse bias analysis and resulting nonresponse-adjusted analysis weights, we determined that estimates using these weights are generalizable to the population of smaller airports and are sufficiently reliable for the purposes of our reporting objectives.

[8] Unless otherwise noted, all estimates from this survey have a margin of error of plus or minus 10 percentage points or less, at the 95 percent confidence level.

To describe the outlook for aviation industry recovery and considerations for the federal role in assisting the aviation industry, we reviewed forecasts published by aviation industry stakeholders, including aviation- related businesses, consulting firms, and credit rating agencies, and synthesized their findings. We also interviewed the 47 aviation and aerospace industry stakeholders described above to obtain their perspectives on considerations for federal assistance, and reviewed our prior work on civil aviation and on federal assistance to the private sector.[9] See appendix I for additional details on our objectives, scope, and methodology, including a list of stakeholders interviewed.

We conducted this performance audit from July 2020 to October 2021 in accordance with generally accepted government auditing standards. Those standards require that we plan and perform the audit to obtain sufficient, appropriate evidence to provide a reasonable basis for our findings and conclusions based on our audit objectives. We believe that the evidence obtained provides a reasonable basis for our findings and conclusions based on our audit objectives.

Background

Civil Aviation and Aerospace Sectors

The U.S. civil aviation and aerospace industries are vital contributors to the domestic and global economies. Airlines generate billions of dollars in revenue annually and contribute to the economic health of the nation. These industries are a complex and dynamic ecosystem that includes, among many other entities, passenger airlines that provide scheduled and non-scheduled service, cargo airlines, airports, aviation manufacturers of airplanes and engines, businesses that provide aircraft maintenance services, and the commercial space industry.[10]

---

[9] See, for example, GAO, *Sustained Federal Action is Crucial as Pandemic Enters Its Second Year,* GAO-21-387 (Washington, D.C.: Mar. 31, 2021), and GAO, *Financial Assistance: Lessons Learned from CARES Act Loan Program for Aviation and Other Eligible Businesses*, GAO-21-198 (Washington, D.C.: Dec. 10, 2020).

[10] Other entities within the industry include businesses that supply various resources to airlines, including catering companies and fuel suppliers; airport tenants such as rental car companies, parking operators, and gift and retail concessionaires; smaller businesses in the aviation manufacturing supply chain, including parts and component suppliers; and business involved in the manufacture and operation of drones.

Passenger Airlines

Airlines that provide scheduled commercial passenger service are often grouped into categories including network, low-cost, and regional airlines. Most network airlines operate complex hub-and-spoke operations with thousands of employees and hundreds of aircraft. These airlines provide service at various levels to a wide variety of domestic and international destinations. Low-cost airlines tend to operate less costly point-to-point service mostly to domestic airports using fewer types of aircraft. Regional airlines operate smaller aircraft, turboprops, or regional jets with up to 100 seats, and generally provide service to smaller communities under capacity purchase agreements with network airlines.[11] Some regional airlines are owned by a network airline, while others are independent. Airlines that provide scheduled commercial passenger service may also carry cargo—called "belly cargo"—in any excess space on the lower decks of their aircraft. Other aircraft operators provide unscheduled, charter, and on-demand passenger service and include air taxis and business jets.[12]

Since the airline industry was deregulated in 1978, its earnings have been volatile.[13] Notably, the demand for air travel tends to fluctuate in relation to the state of the economy as well as to political, international, and health-related events. For example, in the last 20 years, global air travel demand has been disrupted by events including 9/11, the SARS outbreak of 2002-03, and the 2008 global financial crisis. However, airlines experienced a period of sustained profitability from 2010 to 2019 based in part on the strength of the overall economy, consolidation among airlines, and industry's greater ability to align supply with levels of demand.

Airports

The United States has more than 19,000 airports, which vary substantially in size and the type of aviation services they support. Roughly 3,300 are public airports designated by FAA as part of the national airport system,[14] which

[11] Under a capacity purchase agreement, network airlines contract with regional airlines to provide air service beyond the network airline's own route structure to increase their capacity and revenue. Agreement terms vary, but network airlines generally take on all commercial functions, such as brand marketing, flight scheduling, and ticket pricing, while the regional airlines are responsible for the aircraft and crews to operate the flights and provide ground and flight operations.

[12] See 14 C.F.R. pt. 135.

[13] Airline Deregulation Act of 1978, Pub. L. No. 95–504, 92 Stat. 1705.

[14] The 3,300 airports designated by FAA as part of the national airport system are eligible for federal assistance for airport capital projects.

consists of two categories of airports: (1) commercial service, which are publicly owned, have scheduled service, and board at least 2,500 passengers per year, and (2) general aviation and reliever airports, which have either no scheduled service or fewer than 2,500 passengers per year.[15] Federal law divides commercial service airports into various sub-categories, based on the number of passenger boardings (enplanements), ranging from large hub airports to commercial service non-primary airports (see Figure 1).

Airport category	Qualifying percentage range or number of annual passenger enplanements	Percentage of 2018 total U.S. enplanements	Number of U.S. airports
Large hub	1% or more	71%	30
Medium hub	At least 0.25%, but less than 1%	16%	31
Small hub	At least 0.05%, but less than 0.25%	8%	69
Nonhub	More than 10,000, but less than 0.05%	3%	266
Commercial service non-primary	At least 2,500 and no more than 10,000	Not applicable	123

Source: GAO analysis of Federal Aviation Administration (FAA) data. | GAO-22-104429.

Note: Primary commercial service airports are grouped into four hub categories. 49 U.S.C. §§ 47102(11), (13), (14), (25).

Figure 1. Commercial Airport Categories for U.S. Airports.

Commercial service airports collect the bulk of their revenues from two general groups of users: aeronautical users, such as passenger airlines, and non-aeronautical concessionaires, including car rental agencies, parking lots, restaurants, gift shops, and other small vendors. The airports provide these users with a wide range of facilities and services for which they assess fees, rents, or other charges.

Other sectors within the aviation and aerospace industries include:

[15] According to FAA's National Plan of Integrated Airport Systems, 2021-2025, there are 2,535 general aviation airports and 250 reliever airports, which are designated by FAA to relieve congestion at nearby commercial service airports and to provide improved general aviation access to the overall community.

- *Cargo airlines:* This sector includes airlines that operate aircraft configured specifically for carrying cargo. Compared to passenger aircraft that carry some belly cargo, dedicated cargo aircraft can carry more varied types of cargo, such as items that are large or unusually shaped, hazardous material, and livestock and other animals.
- *General aviation:* According to FAA, "general aviation" describes a diverse range of aviation activities and includes all segments of the aviation industry except commercial aviation and the military.[16] General aviation activities include training of new pilots and pilots interested in additional ratings or certification, sightseeing, movement of large heavy loads by helicopter, flying for personal or business/corporate reasons, and emergency medical services. General aviation aircraft range from the one-seat single-engine piston aircraft to the long-range corporate jet, and also include gliders and amateur-built aircraft.
- *Manufacturers:* Airlines purchase commercial aircraft, jet engines, components, and other systems for the global aviation and aerospace industry from an array of manufacturers and related suppliers.
- *Repair station operators:* Three basic types of organizations perform aircraft maintenance for U.S. airlines: (1) airlines' in-house maintenance facilities; (2) original equipment manufacturers (OEMs) that offer maintenance capabilities for the aircraft parts they manufacture; and (3) independent repair stations (i.e., not owned or affiliated in whole or part by airlines or OEMs). Aircraft maintenance services include line maintenance, airframe heavy maintenance, engine repair and overhaul, and component maintenance.[17]
- *Uncrewed aircraft systems:* Uncrewed aircraft systems (UAS), or drones, have the potential to provide significant social and economic benefits in the United States, including by delivering packages, helping to fight fires, and distributing medical supplies at hospitals,

---

[16] FAA, *FAA Aerospace Forecasts, Fiscal Years 2003-2014.*

[17] Line maintenance entails light, regular maintenance checks carried out to ensure that an aircraft is fit for flight. Airframe heavy maintenance involves regularly scheduled inspection, maintenance, preventive maintenance, and alteration that will take aircraft out of service for a pre-determined time at specified intervals. Engine repair and overhaul includes disassembling, inspecting, repairing, or replacing engine parts, followed by reassembling and testing. Component maintenance is the repair and overhaul of components that provide the basic functionality for flight. For more information, see GAO, *Aviation Safety: FAA's Risk-Based Oversight for Repair Stations Could Benefit from Additional Airline Data and Performance Metrics,* GAO-16-679 (Washington, D.C.: July28, 2016).

as well as through military uses, such as intelligence, surveillance, and reconnaissance.[18]

- *Commercial space transportation:* Space transportation is the movement of objects, such as satellites and vehicles carrying cargo, scientific payloads, or passengers, to or from space. In the United States, commercial space transportation is carried out by private companies using orbital and suborbital launch vehicles, which they own and operate.

Federal Assistance to the Aviation Industry during the COVID-19 Pandemic

In response to the public health and economic crises, COVID-19 relief laws have provided more than $100 billion in assistance for aviation businesses and airports since March 2020, and depending on the program, required recipients to temporarily maintain employment levels or refrain from conducting involuntary furloughs, among other requirements.[19] This assistance has included:

- Up to $63 billion in financial assistance to be used exclusively for the continuation of payment of employee wages, salaries, and benefits for eligible applicants including passenger airlines, cargo airlines, and certain aviation contractors;
- Up to $29 billion for loans and loan guarantees to provide liquidity to passenger airlines, cargo airlines, repair stations, and ticket agents;[20]

---

[18] We did not include UAS in the scope of our audit work. In ongoing work, we are examining related issues including, among others, the status of FAA's efforts to integrate UAS into the National Airspace System, federal actions to address the malicious use of UAS in the airport environment, and workforce considerations for the use of UAS in transporting passengers and cargo, or Advanced Air Mobility.

[19] GAO, *COVID-19: Opportunities to Improve Federal Response and Recover Efforts*, GAO-20-625 (Washington, D.C.: June 25, 2020). Conditions of the three financial assistance programs include prohibitions against involuntary layoffs or furloughs. Some airlines took action to offer early retirement. In addition, through attrition and hiring freezes, airlines were able to reduce headcount. As authorized by the CARES Act and the Consolidated Appropriations Act, 2021, DOT required scheduled passenger airlines receiving financial assistance to maintain minimum scheduled passenger service to points in the United States served prior to the pandemic, with some exceptions. Pub. L. No. 116-136, §§ 4005, 4114(b), 134 Stat. at 477, 499; Pub. L. No. 116-260, § 407, 134 Stat. at 2058-59.

[20] CARES Act, § 4003, 134 Stat. at 470. Section 4003 also included up to $17 billion for businesses critical to maintaining national security.

- $20 billion in airport grants to support U.S. airports of all sizes and certain tenants experiencing severe economic disruption caused by the COVID-19 pandemic;[21]
- $3 billion to establish an Aviation Manufacturing Jobs Protection program to provide payroll support payments to eligible businesses exclusively for the continuation of employee wages, salaries, and benefits, and to facilitate the retention, rehire, or recall of employees of the employer;[22] and
- A suspension of aviation excise taxes on air transport of people, cargo, and aviation fuel through calendar year 2020.[23]

The CARES Act provided other assistance for which entities beyond the aviation industry had eligibility, including the Paycheck Protection Program, Main Street Lending Program, and various employer and business tax provisions.[24]

Figure 2 illustrates key trends and events in aviation, public health, and federal assistance during the COVID-19 pandemic in relation to airport traffic and reported COVID-19 infections.

---

[21] Under the Consolidated Appropriations Act, 2021 and the American Rescue Plan Act of 2021, certain amounts were made available to provide relief from rent and minimum annual guarantees to airport concessions. 134 Stat. at 1939-40; § 7102, 135 Stat. at 96-98. The CARES Act gives the FAA the authority to retain up to 0.1 percent of the $10 billion (equaling up to $10 million) provided for Grants-in-Aid for Airports to fund the award and oversight by FAA of grants made under the CARES Act. Pub. L. No. 116-136, 134 Stat. at 596-597.

[22] Under the American Rescue Plan Act of 2021, DOT may use up to 1 percent of the funds appropriated ($30 million) for implementation costs and administrative expenses. Pub. L. No. 117-2 § 7202(a), 135 Stat. at 103.

[23] In October 2020, Congress appropriated $14 billion from the General Fund to the Airport and Airway Trust Fund, the income of which had been affected by reduced revenues from air travel during the pandemic and the CARES Act's suspension of aviation excise taxes. Continuing Appropriations Act, 2021 and Other Extensions Act, Pub. L. No. 116-159, § 1205, 134 Stat. 709, 728. The Trust Fund funds, among other things, federal grants for airports, acquisition and maintenance for air traffic facilities and equipment, and research on issues related to aviation safety, mobility, and technologies. The Trust Fund receives income from sources including taxes on airline passenger ticket sales, segment fees, air cargo fees, and aviation fuel taxes paid by both commercial and general aviation aircraft.

[24] For a broader discussion of these COVID-19 relief provisions, see GAO, *COVID-19: Continued Attention Needed to Enhance Federal Preparedness, Response, Service Delivery, and Program Integrity*, GAO-21-551 (Washington, D.C.: July 19, 2021).

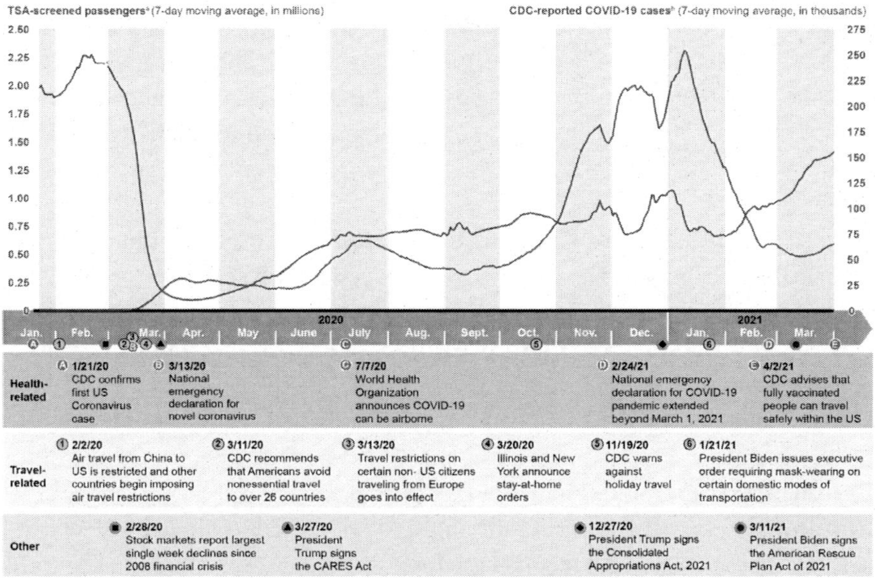

Source: GAO analysis of Transportation Security Administration (TSA) information, Centers for Disease Control and Prevention (CDC) information, COVID-19 relief laws and Presidential documents, and Reuters news reports. | GAO-22-104429.

Notes:

[a]TSA screened passenger data include TSA, airport, and airline employees transiting checkpoints and therefore represents slightly more than actual passenger traffic. The 7-day moving averages were calculated as the (current day + 6 preceding days)/7, where data were reported. The TSA data were accessed on August 31, 2021.

[b]Reported COVID-19 cases include confirmed and probable cases. The 7-day moving averages were calculated as the (current day + 6 preceding days)/7, where data were reported. The CDC data were accessed on August 27, 2021.

[c]The TSA screened passenger data on February 29, 2020 was not reported and therefore not included in the 7-day moving average.

Figure 2. TSA-Screened Passengers, CDC-Reported COVID-19 Cases, and Selected Key Events during the COVID-19 Pandemic (January 2020 through March 2021).

The COVID-19 Pandemic Had Disparate Effects on Selected Aviation and Aerospace Sectors in 2020

The COVID-19 pandemic had disparate effects on selected aviation and aerospace sectors in 2020, most severely affecting the sectors that are dependent on commercial passenger activity. The dramatic drop in demand for passenger air travel had a cascading effect across commercial aviation sectors, including passenger airlines, airports, aviation manufacturers, and repair station operators. However, other aviation and aerospace sectors that are less reliant on passenger activity, such as cargo airlines, business aviation, and the commercial space transportation industry, experienced less of a reduction—and in some cases an increase—in demand for their services.

The Dramatic Drop in Demand for Passenger Air Travel in 2020 Had Cascading Effects across Commercial Aviation Sectors

Passenger Airlines Experienced Unprecedented Reduction in Demand for Air Travel

U.S. passenger airlines experienced an unprecedented reduction in the demand for air travel in 2020 as a result of the COVID-19 pandemic. According to Bureau of Transportation Statistics (BTS) data, annual airline passenger traffic was down 60 percent system-wide in 2020 compared to annual traffic levels in 2019. Passenger traffic reached the lowest levels in April 2020, when traffic fell to 3 million passengers, a 96 percent decrease compared to the previous April. As the industry group Airlines for America (A4A) testified to Congress, such low traffic levels had not been seen since the 1950s.[25]

Passenger traffic has slowly returned since the trough in demand in April 2020, with the return of domestic traffic outpacing the return of international traffic (see Figure 3). Annual international air traffic was over 70 percent lower in 2020 compared to 2019 and accounted for 9 percent of all U.S. passenger air traffic, compared to 12 percent in 2019.

In addition, business passengers have been slower to return than leisure passengers. This slower return is in part due to the increased use of virtual meeting technology, according to the consulting firm McKinsey & Company,[26] as well as potential liability concerns. According to data collected by the Airlines Reporting Corporation (ARC), the sale of corporate tickets reached its lowest point in April 2020 when sales were down over 96 percent from the prior year. ARC data further indicates that sales of corporate tickets remained low throughout 2020, continuing to be approximately 80 percent lower than pre-pandemic levels as of late December 2020.

---

[25] *Prepare for Takeoff: America's Safe Return to Air Travel, Hearing on SR-253, Before the U.S. Senate Committee on Commerce, Science, and Transportation Subcommittee on Aviation Safety, Operations, and Innovation*, 117th Cong. (2021) (statement of Nick Calio, President and CEO, Airlines for America).

[26] McKinsey & Company, *For Corporate travel, a long recovery ahead* (August 2020).

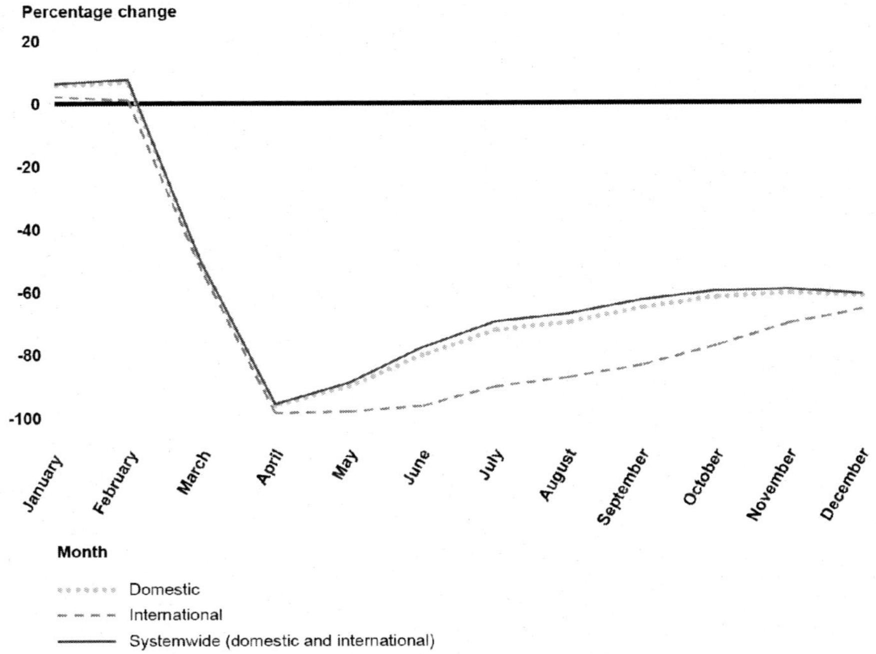

Source: GAO analysis of Department of Transportation Bureau of Transportation Statistics data. | GAO-22-104429.

Figure 3. U.S. Airline Passenger Traffic, Percentage Change 2019 versus 2020, by Type.

This sharp decline in demand affected airlines' revenues, but the extent of that effect varied across airlines based on their business models.

- *Network airlines:* The long period of reduced business and international passenger traffic has particularly affected the revenues of network airlines, which typically generate a large portion of their revenues from such travelers. According to the credit rating agency Moody's, large U.S. network airlines generate at least one third of their revenue from business travelers, despite the fact that business travelers make up only about 12 percent of global passengers.[27] Based on BTS data, Delta Air Lines, American Airlines, and United Airlines—the top three major U.S. network airlines based on 2019 operating revenues—experienced a 94 percent decline in passenger

[27] Moody's Investors Service, *Business Travel Faces Higher Substitution Risk post- COVID, but Airlines will Adapt* (Mar. 24, 2021).

revenues in the second quarter of 2020 compared to the second quarter of 2019.[28] By the fourth quarter of 2020, the three network airlines' passenger revenues remained down 76 percent. While the decline in revenues was largely due to the decline in passengers, fare reductions also had an effect. For example, selected network airlines reduced their gross average fare by 19 percent in 2020 compared to 2019, in part to attract passenger traffic.[29] For the majority of the year, these airlines were experiencing negative cash flow or "cash burn," whereby they needed to use cash reserves to fund their daily operations. For example, United Airlines reported that it spent $40 million more per day than it earned in revenue in the second quarter of 2020.

- *Low-cost airlines:* Low-cost airlines' business models rely largely on customers flying domestically for leisure travel at generally lower airfares than those charged by network airlines. These airlines experienced a faster return of their passenger traffic, and in turn their revenues, than network airlines. For example, according to BTS data, six selected low-cost airlines experienced an 87 percent decline in passenger revenues in the second quarter of 2020 compared to 2019.[30] By the fourth quarter of 2020, the low-cost airlines' passenger revenues were down only 67 percent compared to the same quarter in the prior year. Like network airlines, low-cost airlines' revenues were also affected by their fare reductions. Selected low-cost airlines reduced their average gross fare by 21 percent in 2020 compared to 2019. Low-cost airlines also experienced negative cash flow, but recovered faster than the network airlines. For example, Spirit Airlines reported that it spent approximately $9.5 million more per day than it earned in revenue in April 2020, but in the fourth quarter—October through December—of 2020 it reduced that daily average negative cash flow to $1.8 million.
- *Regional airlines:* Regional airlines, whose business models rely on contracts with their network airline partners, experienced mixed impacts from the pandemic. Four regional airlines ceased operation

---

[28] Passenger revenue is revenue received by the airline from the carriage of passengers in scheduled operations.

[29] Gross fare was calculated using U.S. DOT Origin & Destination summary data, which sources from a 10% sample of all U.S. airline tickets.

[30] Based on BTS 2019 airline rankings of the top 21 airlines by operating revenue, we included Allegiant Air, Frontier Airlines, JetBlue Airways, Southwest Airlines, Spirit Airlines, and Sun Country Airlines in our analysis of low-cost airlines.

in 2020; however, certain remaining regional airlines were profitable in 2020 due to the nature of their existing contracts with their network airline partners. For example, representatives from one regional airline we interviewed credited their profitability in 2020 in part to the fact that their business is based primarily on what are called "capacity purchase agreements." Under these agreements, network airline partners contract with regional airlines to provide service on regional routes, and in exchange, the network airlines generally pay a variety of the regional airlines' costs, including, for example, a guaranteed monthly fee and payment for the regional airlines' hours in service and certain other flight costs such as fuel. Additionally, representatives from another regional airline told us that in some cases, they flew flights on routes on which their network airline partners previously flew larger jets, as their network airline partners responded to decreased demand by flying smaller, less expensive regional aircraft on certain routes instead of mostly empty, larger jets.

Airport Revenues Declined as a Result of Reduced Demand for Air Travel

U.S. airports experienced a significant reduction in passenger traffic as a result of the pandemic, although the extent of this reduction varied depending on the type of travelers an airport typically serves. Large airports that serve business and international travelers—such as JFK International Airport and Boston Logan International Airport—experienced a greater and more sustained decline in passenger traffic compared to airports that are in leisure destinations. For example, according to data from A4A, traveler throughput in New York and Massachusetts was down more than 75 percent in November 2020 compared to November 2019, while Florida and Arizona—which are popular U.S. leisure travel destinations—experienced declines of approximately 50 percent over the same period.

Based on our interviews with large and medium hub airport representatives and our survey of smaller airports, we found that airports of all sizes experienced a decline in both aeronautical[31] and non- aeronautical

[31] The estimated percentage (lower bound, upper bound) of airports reporting a decline in aeronautical revenue between September 2019 and September 2020 was 85 (73, 93) percent for small hub airports, 92 (87, 96) percent for non-hub airports, 69 (56, 80) percent for non-primary commercial service airports, and 54 (50, 58) percent for general aviation and reliever airports. The margins of error between the estimates for the small hub and non-primary commercial service airports and the upper or lower bounds were greater than 10 percentage points. These estimates should be interpreted with caution.

operating revenues as a result of the COVID-19 pandemic.[32] Specifically, representatives from the large and medium hub airports we interviewed reported that their revenue losses were tied to decreases in the various forms of passenger-driven operating revenues they collect. For example, representatives at one large hub airport told us that relative to 2019 levels, aeronautical operating revenue collected from landing fees paid by airlines at their airport was down approximately 60 percent in April 2020 and down 30 percent in September 2020. Furthermore, representatives from some of these airports told us that passenger-driven sources of non-aeronautical revenues such as concessions and parking had dropped 35 percent or more in 2020 compared to 2019.

Similarly, based on the smaller airports we surveyed, we estimate that small hub and non-hub airports experienced greater percentage declines in revenues than non-primary commercial service or general aviation and reliever airports,[33] a reflection of the small- and non-hub airports' heavier reliance on scheduled commercial passenger service. For example, based on our survey, we estimate that about 60 percent of all smaller airports had a decrease in aeronautical revenues in September 2020 compared to September 2019, and among those airports, about a quarter experienced a decrease in revenues of more than 50 percent. Additionally, we estimate that about half of small hub and about one-third of non-hub airports experienced a decrease in non-aeronautical revenues of more than 50 percent. At the same time,

---

[32] Airports generate both aeronautical revenues and non-aeronautical revenues. Aeronautical revenues are derived from the operation and landing of aircraft, passengers, or freight. As discussed later, airports assess fees on airlines for the use of the airport based on negotiated agreements. These agreements vary in whether the airline or the airport bears the risk if the fees paid by airlines and others do not fully cover the airport's costs. Non-aeronautical revenues are derived from sources unrelated to the operation and landing of aircraft, passengers, or freight, such as terminal concessions and parking fees.

[33] The estimated percentage (lower bound, upper bound) of airports reporting a decline in aeronautical revenue of more than 50 percent between September 2019 and September 2020 was 30 (19, 44) percent for small hub airports, 38 (36, 41) percent for non-hub airports, 15 (7, 26) percent for non-primary commercial service airports, and 12 (9, 15) percent for general aviation and reliever airports. The margins of error between the estimates for the small hub and non-primary commercial service airports and the upper or lower bounds were greater than 10 percentage points. These estimates should be interpreted with caution. The estimated percentage (lower bound, upper bound) of airports reporting a decline in non-aeronautical revenue of more than 50 percent between September 2019 and September 2020 was 47 (44, 51) percent for small hub airports, 32 (30, 34) percent for non-hub airports, 13 (6, 24) percent for non-primary commercial service airports, and 7 (5, 9) percent for general aviation and reliever airports. The margins of error between the estimates for the non-primary commercial service airports and the upper or lower bounds were greater than 10 percentage points. These estimates should be interpreted with caution.

however, about 60 percent of general aviation and reliever airports and about 40 percent of non-primary commercial service airports did not see a change in their non- aeronautical revenues. For the full results of our survey of smaller airports, see appendix II.

Declining Passenger Travel Led to Reduced Demand for Commercial Airplanes, Engines, and Aircraft Maintenance Services

In response to reduced passenger demand, airlines parked or retired a substantial portion of their aircraft fleet (as we discuss later in this report), which in turn reduced demand for new commercial airplanes, engines, and spare parts in the near term. According to representatives we interviewed from two aviation manufacturers and one supplier, and financial statements publicly reported by these businesses, they experienced a decline in revenues as a result of delayed delivery or deferred orders from airlines and other manufacturers. For example, one large engine manufacturer publicly reported that its aviation segment orders were down $15.1 billion—41 percent—in 2020 compared to 2019. It attributed the decrease primarily to lower commercial equipment and service orders as airline customers slowed or deferred new engine orders. For these manufacturers, the effects of the pandemic were preceded by the financial impact of the 737 MAX grounding in 2019, which affected not only Boeing but companies in the supply chain that produced components for the 737 MAX.[34]

Airline decisions in response to passenger demand also affected businesses that provide aircraft maintenance services. Representatives from three repair station operators told us that airline decisions to reduce capacity by flying less frequently reduced demand for maintenance services in the near term. For example, representatives from one repair station operator reported that demand from their commercial airline customers declined by 70-80 percent. Additionally, according to a June 2020 survey by the Aeronautical Repair Station Association, 87 percent of member repair station respondents reported revenue declines in January–May 2020, with an average decline of about 46 percent.[35]

---

[34] On March 13, 2019, FAA issued an emergency order prohibiting the operation of Boeing 737 MAX series aircraft by U.S. certificated operators in response to the crashes of Lion Air Flight 610 in Indonesia on October 28, 2018 and Ethiopian Airlines Flight 302 on March 10, 2019. FAA rescinded the emergency order and cleared the MAX to fly again on November 18, 2020.

[35] Aeronautical Repair Station Association, "Pandemic Impacts on Aviation Markets: Employment and Revenue Losses Reported by U.S. Maintenance Companies, January 1, 2020 to June 1, 2020," July 28, 2020.

Other Aviation and Aerospace Sectors Experienced Increased Demand or Suffered a Less Severe Reduction in Demand in 2020

Cargo Airlines

As a result of the larger number of people staying home during the pandemic and the growth in e-commerce, domestic cargo airlines experienced an increased demand for service. According to BTS data, 2020 was a record year in the amount of cargo carried by airlines. In 2020, the top fifteen U.S. airlines based on tons of cargo transported in 2020 carried 1.46 million more tons of cargo than in 2019, an increase of 10.7 percent year-over-year.[36] These airlines experienced an average 5.5 percent increase in total operating revenues in 2020 compared to 2019.

Representatives from the large cargo airline we spoke with told us that in the early stage of the pandemic, neither their company nor the broader U.S. cargo aviation system had the capacity to meet the quick increase in demand for cargo services; however, the industry was able to accommodate this increase in demand relatively quickly. The decrease in passenger airline flights reduced cargo capacity early in the pandemic because passenger flights normally carry some cargo in the belly of their aircraft. However, capacity constraints were eased as passenger airlines' traffic picked up and as some cargo was accommodated on empty passenger planes. Additionally, representatives from the large cargo airline we spoke with told us they also met the increased demand for cargo transport in part by ramping up their hiring of 100,000 winter-season employees earlier in the year than usual and maintaining those workforce levels through the winter.

Representatives from the two smaller charter cargo airlines we spoke with told us they experienced uncertainty and volatility in their operations in 2020. Representatives told us that they initially experienced large decreases in demand early in 2020 as the markets they served shut down, starting with China in January and February, followed by Europe and then the U.S. in March. As a result, representatives from both airlines told us that in the first quarter of 2020, they were losing money and under financial stress. However, they told us they experienced a return in demand as the markets they service reopened, starting in mid-to-late spring 2020.

[36] The largest fifteen cargo airlines were based on total freight and mail transported in 2020. These airlines generated at least 30 percent of their operating revenues from freight and mail transport.

Business Aviation

Similar to other aviation sectors, business aviation— the use of smaller, general aviation aircraft primarily for business purposes—experienced a steep decline in activity early in the pandemic; however, demand began to recover for this sector in the second half of 2020, much faster than for passenger airlines. For example, according to FAA data, domestic and international business jet operations in April 2020 were nearly 75 percent below 2019 levels, but by June 2020 had recovered to levels 24 percent below those in June 2019, and by December 2020 were only about 12 percent lower than the prior year's level of activity.[37] According to a December 2020 report from S&P Global Ratings, demand for business aviation had rebounded in part due to increased demand from corporate executives and individuals able to pay for alternatives to commercial scheduled passenger service during the pandemic.[38]

Representatives from the two business jet manufacturers we interviewed reported decreased demand in spring 2020 as a result of the pandemic, but told us that demand improved in the latter half of the year. They attributed lower demand in part to customer uncertainty concerning the timing of economic recovery and managing supply chain disruptions. In particular, both manufacturers told us that domestic and global travel restrictions presented challenges in completing aircraft deliveries; however, they told us it was helpful that customers generally delayed or deferred aircraft orders rather than cancel them altogether. Both manufacturers experienced increased demand for their products in the third and fourth quarters of 2020 compared to the first half of the year. Officials from one manufacturer we spoke with attributed this improvement to a combination of increased optimism around vaccine availability and distribution, a better understanding of how the pandemic may progress, and general optimism about the direction of the economy. According to shipment data for U.S. manufactured aircraft from the General Aviation Manufacturers Association, whose membership includes business jet manufacturers, deliveries of business jets increased in the third and fourth quarters of 2020 versus the first half of the year, but overall were 12 percent lower in 2020 than in 2019.

---

[37] Federal Aviation Administration, *Business Jet Report: January 2021.*

[38] S&P Global Ratings, *Industry Top Trends 2021: Aerospace and Defense* (Dec.10, 2020).

Commercial Space Transportation

Representatives we spoke with from the commercial space transportation industry told us that, to date, the COVID-19 pandemic has had varied effects on the industry. Some sectors of commercial space transportation experienced growth—namely the commercial space launch sector that, while largely driven by one launch provider, experienced a 50 percent increase in the number of FAA-licensed commercial launches from calendar year 2019 to 2020.[39] Representatives from an industry association and an analytics and engineering firm told us that the demand for some sectors of commercial space dropped—such as demand for satellite services to commercial airlines and cruise ships. However, representatives from an industry association explained that because commercial space companies generally have longer-range business models than traditional aviation, a decrease in demand does not immediately affect the sustainability of operations.

Aviation and Aerospace Stakeholders Responded to the Pandemic's Effects by Taking a Variety of Actions to Maintain Business Viability

In response to the many effects of the COVID-19 pandemic, aviation stakeholders reported that throughout 2020, they quickly implemented measures to mitigate financial losses and position themselves to maintain business viability until demand recovers.[40] These actions included managing costs—which often included reducing costs; using federal assistance provided through COVID-19 relief legislation; raising funds in the private market; and taking actions to mitigate the spread of COVID-19 among employees and customers.

---

[39] We have previously reported on the growth and evolution of the commercial space transportation industry and FAA's efforts to oversee it. See, for example, GAO, *Commercial Space Transportation: FAA Continues to Update Regulations and Faces Challenges to Overseeing an Evolving Industry,* GAO-21-105268 (Washington, D.C.: June 16, 2021); *Commercial Space Transportation: FAA Should Examine a Range of Options to Support U.S. Launch Infrastructure*, GAO-21-154 (Washington, D.C.: Dec. 22, 2020); and *Commercial Space Transportation: Improvements to FAA's Workforce Planning Needed to Prepare for the Industry's Anticipated Growth,* GAO-19-437 (Washington, D.C.: May 23, 2019).

[40] We excluded from this discussion commercial space transportation for which the pandemic had less deleterious effects.

Aviation and Aerospace Stakeholders Took Several Actions to Manage Labor and Other Operating Costs, and Reduced Capital Investments

Labor Costs

Passenger airlines took several actions to manage labor costs throughout 2020, such as offering employees voluntary unpaid leave or separation and early retirement programs, freezing non-essential hiring, and implementing involuntary furloughs within the limits of the COVID-19 relief laws.[41] For example, Delta Air Lines reported in public SEC financial reports that 50,000 employees took voluntary unpaid leaves of absence and approximately 18,000 employees participated in the airline's early retirement and voluntary separation programs in 2020. American Airlines reported reducing its management and support staff team by approximately 5,100 positions (30 percent) in 2020 and that more than 20,000 of its employees opted for early retirement or long-term partially paid leave as of December 2020. Furthermore, American Airlines, Delta Air Lines, and United Airlines all reported freezing non-essential hiring.

Airports took similar actions to manage their labor costs throughout 2020, although only a small percentage of workers at U.S. airports are employed by the airport.[42] Airports that accepted grant funds from the federal COVID-19 relief programs were also limited in their ability to reduce employment levels or conduct involuntary furloughs.[43] Representatives from nearly all of the eleven large and medium hub airports we spoke with cited managing costs through suspending or slowing down hiring. For example, representatives at one large hub airport operated by a municipal government told us their airport was affected by a hiring slow-down that limited new hiring to only critical

---

[41] Aviation stakeholders across sectors reduced labor costs. However, as discussed above, airlines and airports accepting federal assistance from the CARES Act and subsequent COVID-19 relief laws were limited in their ability to reduce employment levels or conduct involuntary furloughs.

[42] Airport direct hires are a small number of people who work at an airport. Many people working in airports are employees of private companies, such as airlines and airport tenants. For example, gate agents are hired by airlines and concessionaire employees are hired directly by concessionaires.

[43] Certain airport owners—also known as airport sponsors—accepting CARES Act grant funds were required to continue to employ, through December 31, 2020, at least 90 percent of the number of individuals employed as of March 27, 2020. However, non-hub and non-primary airports were excluded from this workforce retention requirement. The Consolidated Appropriations Act, 2021 extended these workforce retention requirements through February 15, 2021. Airports that accept American Rescue Plan Act of 2021 grants will be subject to the same workforce retention requirements through September 30, 2021.

positions. In addition, representatives from four airports we spoke with told us they offered voluntary early retirement programs. Representatives from one of the eleven airports we spoke with told us they went through a reduction in force limited to 26 union and non-union employees, which reduced the airport's payroll by about 5 percent. Based on our survey of smaller airports, we estimate that about 5 percent of smaller airports implemented staff layoffs and about 20 percent of smaller airports decreased staff hours to reduce operating costs at their airports.

Representatives from two manufacturers and two repair station operators we interviewed also reported that they reduced their workforces in 2020 through reductions to employees' hours, layoffs, furloughs, and in some cases, closing facilities. For example, representatives from one repair station operator that did not receive COVID-19 relief funding told us they reduced their staff by 50 percent in 2020. Similarly, one large manufacturer of airplane engines permanently reduced its global workforce of 52,000 employees by approximately 25 percent in 2020, and representatives from a business jet manufacturer told us that more than 600 employees were affected in October 2020 when it decided to permanently close a facility in California.[44]

Non-Labor Operating and Capital Investments

Passenger airlines also took a number of actions in 2020 to manage non- labor operating costs and certain capital investments. Early on in the pandemic, some passenger airlines took actions to better align supply with demand by quickly reducing the capacity and reach of their networks. They did this by reducing flight frequencies, the number of airports they served, and the size of aircraft flying certain routes (including shifting flights to regional airlines), which reduced operating costs; however, the extent to which they were able to reduce service was limited in some cases.[45] The three selected network airlines included in our earlier analysis—Delta Air Lines, American Airlines, and United Airlines— reduced system-wide capacity, as measured in available

---

[44] Neither manufacturer received CARES Act assistance and were therefore not limited in their ability to reduce employment levels.

[45] As authorized by the CARES Act and the Consolidated Appropriations Act, 2021, DOT required scheduled passenger airlines receiving financial assistance to maintain minimum scheduled passenger service to points in the United States served prior to the pandemic, with some exceptions, until March 1, 2022. For example, DOT has exempted airlines in cases where it is not reasonable or practicable to serve all points or all frequencies in their service obligations. Pub. L. No. 116-136, §§ 4005, 4114(b), 134 Stat. at 477, 499; Pub. L. No. 116-260, § 407, 134 Stat. at 2058-59.

seat miles, by 54 percent in 2020 compared to 2019 levels.[46] The six selected low-cost airlines reduced system-wide capacity by 37 percent during the same time period.

Additionally, airlines also reduced costs by retiring older aircraft, delaying the delivery of new aircraft, or both, in an effort to reduce both operating and capital costs. According to FAA data, U.S. mainline carriers reduced the number of passenger jet aircraft in their fleet by an estimated 28 percent in 2020.[47] For example, American Airlines accelerated the retirement of a number of aircraft, including certain Airbus A330, Boeing 757 and Boeing 767 models, and certain regional aircraft. According to American's SEC financial reports, the aircraft retirements provided cost savings and efficiencies associated with operating fewer aircraft types. Several airlines also placed some aircraft in temporary storage to reduce operating costs (see Figure 4). Some airlines also reduced capital costs by delaying and deferring the delivery of new aircraft, including those scheduled for delivery in 2020 and 2021.

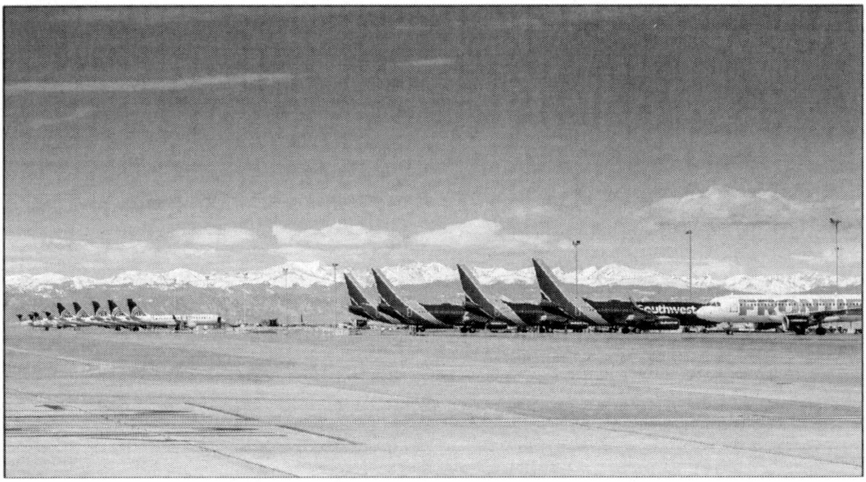

Source: Denver International Airport. | GAO-22-104429.

Figure 4. Parked Aircraft Temporarily Stored at Denver International Airport.

---

[46] Available seat miles are a measure of airline output that refers to one aircraft seat flown one mile, whether occupied or not.

[47] FAA defines mainline carriers as those providing service primarily via aircraft with 90 or more seats.

Airports of all sizes also took actions in 2020 to manage non-labor operating costs and capital investments. For example, representatives from one medium hub airport told us they closed parking lots and reduced shuttle services to cut operating expenses. Additionally, representatives from airports we interviewed and surveyed reported changing the timeline of capital development projects. Representatives from one medium hub airport told us the airport paused a $1.5 billion expansion project that includes the addition of 16 new gates, a seven-story parking garage, a new cargo facility, and several other improvements to the airport. At the same time, representatives from four airports we interviewed told us they accelerated the timeline of some of their capital projects to take advantage of project savings that could be realized as a result of the reduced passenger traffic. Similarly, based on our survey of smaller airports, we estimate that about one third of smaller airports modified their infrastructure project timelines. Among smaller airports that made changes to their infrastructure projects, we estimate that about 15 percent of them cancelled projects and about 75 percent of them delayed projects, while approximately 10 percent accelerated projects.[48]

Representatives from manufacturers and repair station operators told us that they also took actions to manage operating and capital costs in response to reduced demand for commercial and business aircraft, engines, and other aviation components and associated maintenance services throughout 2020. Representatives from several aircraft manufacturers told us they reduced spending on things such as research and development, marketing, advertising, and capital expenditures. Representatives from three repair station operators told us they closed facilities, delayed previously planned expansions, or deferred other capital expenditures as demand for their services decreased.

Aviation Stakeholders Used Federal Assistance Programs to Mitigate Financial Losses

Passenger Airlines Leveraged a Variety of Assistance Programs

To help offset losses and maintain business viability, passenger airlines leveraged federal assistance that, among other things, subsidized employee payroll, provided liquidity, and made changes to tax provisions. Up to $40 billion in financial assistance payments was made available for passenger

---

[48] These numbers are not mutually exclusive—one airport could have multiple projects, some of which were delayed or cancelled, and others of which were accelerated.

airlines by the two rounds of the Payroll Support Program (PSP) established in COVID-19 relief legislation passed in 2020 and another $14 billion in the third round of PSP established in legislation passed in 2021.[49] According to data from Department of the Treasury (Treasury), 354 first-round PSP and 302 second-round PSP agreements were signed with passenger airlines for financial assistance payments that totaled about $39.7 billion as of August 2021. The CARES Act also authorized Treasury to provide up to $29 billion for loans and loan guarantees to provide liquidity to passenger airlines, cargo airlines, repair stations, and ticket agents.[50] Treasury executed loans that allowed 24 aviation-related businesses to bridge revenue declines and pay for ongoing expenses, including payroll and rent; the majority of the loan funds approved—$20.8 billion of a total $21.2 billion—were for seven major passenger airlines.[51] In addition, representatives from airlines reported using the tax provisions in the CARES Act[52]—which included, among other things, an employee retention credit and a delay in payment of employer payroll taxes—to bolster their liquidity. Furthermore, commercial aviation operators also benefited from a CARES Act provision suspending certain commercial air transportation taxes, including those on passenger tickets, cargo, and fuel.[53]

---

[49] As a condition of accepting financial assistance under the Payroll Support Program, Treasury required passenger airlines receiving more than $100 million and contractors receiving more than $37.5 million to provide warrants or notes as taxpayer protection. The American Rescue Plan Act of 2021 was enacted on March 11, 2021, and included a third round of the Payroll Support Program. As of August 2021, Treasury was continuing to sign agreements for assistance from the American Rescue Plan Act of 2021.

[50] CARES Act, § 4003, 134 Stat. at 470. Section 4003 also included up to $17 billion for businesses critical to maintaining national security; however, no aviation businesses applied for this assistance.

[51] As of August 1, 2021, seven aviation-related businesses had fully repaid their loans, including six passenger airlines, as discussed later in this report. These seven loans have a total authorized value of $18.3 billion. GAO has reviewed the implementation of the loan program, including the impacts on both recipients and non-recipients, in prior work; smaller businesses did not see the same benefits from the funds as large passenger airlines. See: GAO, *COVID-19: Continued Attention Needed to Enhance Federal Preparedness, Response, Service Delivery, and Program Integrity*, GAO-21-551 (Washington, D.C.: July 19, 2021); *COVID-19: Sustained Federal Action is Crucial as Pandemic Enters Its Second Year*, GAO-21-387 (Washington, D.C.: March 31, 2021); *Financial Assistance: Lessons Learned from CARES Act Loan Program for Aviation and Other Eligible Businesses,* GAO-20-198 (Washington, D.C.: December 10, 2020); *COVID- 19: Federal Efforts Could Be Strengthened by Timely and Concerted Actions*, GAO-20-701 (Washington, D.C.: September 21, 2021); and *COVID-19: Opportunities to Improve Federal Response and Recovery Efforts,* GAO-20-625 (Washington, D.C.: June 25, 2020).

[52] CARES Act, §§ 2301, 2302, 134 Stat. at 347-52.

[53] CARES Act, § 4007, 134 Stat. at 477.

Representatives from passenger airlines and credit rating agencies told us that federal assistance was essential to cover airline passenger expenses, keep employees on their payrolls, and help stem cash outflows while passenger traffic levels were at historic lows. Representatives from four airlines told us that the PSP program, in particular, provided critical and timely support. For instance, representatives from two airlines emphasized that the PSP program prevented furloughs that would have resulted in employees filing unemployment claims and losing their health care benefits. Representatives from one network airline told us that the loans from Treasury also provided liquidity that was vital for them to continue to operate and maintain their infrastructure until passenger demand returned. The tax-related provisions had a smaller effect on airlines than PSP assistance, but representatives from two credit rating agencies noted that the provisions helped stem airlines' cash outflows.[54] For example, according to SEC financial reports, United Airlines elected to defer the payment of $199 million in payroll taxes incurred through December 31, 2020, and will pay half in December 2021 and the remaining balance in December 2022.

Airports Leveraged Flexible Federal Assistance to Make Debt and Other Payments and Provide Assistance to Airlines and Tenants

According to our interviews, the results of our survey, and our previous reporting on federal COVID-19 assistance programs, airports of all sizes leveraged the flexibility of the federal grants provided for COVID-19 relief to make necessary debt and other payments and provide assistance to airlines and other airport tenants.[55] These federal grants of up to $20 billion in total allowed airports to respond to the COVID-19 pandemic, including funding their operations and meeting their ongoing debt payments, although the funding allocation and allowable uses for the grants differ under the CARES Act and subsequent COVID-19 relief laws.[56] FAA has begun to collect data

---

[54] Airlines and aviation manufacturers reported using tax provisions of the CARES Act, including deferring employer payroll taxes, claiming employee retention credits, and carrying back five years net operating losses arising in tax years beginning in 2018, 2019, and 2020. Pub. L. No. 116-136, §§ 2301-2303, 134 Stat. at 347-56. The Consolidated Appropriations Act, 2021 made a number of changes to these provisions, including extending the availability of credits, among other changes. Pub. L. No. 116-260, div. N, §§ 206-207, 134 Stat. at 3059-65.

[55] GAO-21-551.

[56] The CARES Act, the Consolidated Appropriations Act, 2021, and the American Rescue Plan Act of 2021 provide a combined total of $20 billion in federal funding for U.S. airports to respond to the COVID-19 pandemic. As of May 14, 2021, of the $20 billion, about $10.6 billion has been obligated and $6.5 billion expended by FAA. Under the CARES Act, funds

from airports on general spending categories for the federal COVID-19 relief funding, but officials said that they will have limited information until airports draw down all funds for reimbursed costs.[57]

In our interviews, representatives from large and medium hub airports told us they appreciated the flexibility they had to use the CARES Act grant funding. Representatives from six large and medium hub airports told us they prioritized using the funds for routine, large expenses such as debt service payments and payroll. Representatives from one of these airports specified that they prioritized large expenses because they were among the easiest to have reimbursed by FAA. Three told us they also used the CARES Act grant funding to provide indirect relief to concessionaires such as gift shops and restaurants.[58] In addition, representatives from four large and medium hub airports told us they used the funding to avoid increasing rates they charge airlines. Airports assess fees on airlines for the use of the airport based on negotiated agreements. These agreements vary in whether the airline or the airport bears the risk if the fees paid by airlines and others do not fully cover the airport's costs. In cases where the agreement requires the airlines to make up the difference, the dramatic fall in traffic meant that fees paid by airlines would have had to rise to cover the shortfall. Representatives from large and medium hub airports with such agreements told us they applied CARES Act grant funding to certain costs to airlines to keep fees paid by airlines for

were available for any purpose for which airport revenues may lawfully be used. Underthe Consolidated Appropriations Act, 2021 and the American Rescue Plan of 2021, funds were generally available for costs related to operations, personnel, cleaning, sanitization, janitorial services, combating the spread of pathogens at the airport, and debt service payments. According to FAA guidance, examples of eligible development to combat the spread of pathogens at the airport include replacing or upgrading a heating, ventilation, and air conditioning system, and reconfiguring the terminal to accommodate increased social distancing or health screening. Additionally, under the Consolidated Appropriations Act, 2021 and the American Rescue Plan Act of 2021, certain amounts were made available to provide relief from rent and minimum annual guarantees to airport concessions.

57 FAA has begun to collect and consolidate data from airports on general spending categories for CARES Act funding through grant close-out reports, which are completed once all allocated airport funds have been expended. As of May 14, 2021, FAA officials said that 476 CARES Act airport grants, totaling $1.66 billion, have been closed out. For these grants, the majority of airport grant funds have been used for debt service (about 52 percent of these funds, totaling $864 million) and payroll (about 39 percent of these funds, totaling $643 million). While FAA continues to collect these data on airport grant spending, officials said airports are generally using CARES Act funds on payroll, utilities, minor maintenance, and debt service.

58 The Consolidated Appropriations Act, 2021 and American Rescue Plan Act of 2021 appropriated funds for sponsors of primary airports to provide relief from rent and minimum annual guarantees to on-airport car rental, on-airport parking, and in-terminal airport concessions.

landing and terminal rentals flat, when otherwise fees would have had to rise due to decreased traffic.

Based on our survey of smaller airports, we estimate that about 90 percent of smaller airports received a CARES Act Airport Grant. Of those, about half used the funds for payroll and labor expenses. When asked to describe ways in which the CARES Act worked well in providing support, 87 airports specifically noted that the CARES Act allowed them to avoid either layoffs, furloughs of staff, or both. Smaller airports also used the funds for utilities, equipment, and debt service. Furthermore, we estimate that about one-quarter of smaller airports, and disproportionately small hub and non-hub airports, provided rent or other relief to their tenants,[59] such as deferring payments, waiving payments, and changing or adjusting lease agreements.[60]

Other Aviation and Aerospace Stakeholders Also Leveraged Federal Assistance

Several other aviation and aerospace stakeholders leveraged federal assistance, although the assistance they received was smaller in magnitude than that provided to passenger airlines and airports. For example:

- *Manufacturers:* Representatives from one manufacturer told us they used tax provisions in the CARES Act to bolster the company's liquidity, and another manufacturer reported taking similar action.[61] For example, one manufacturer reported using the 5-year net

---

[59] The estimated percentage (lower bound, upper bound) of airports reporting having provided any rent or other relief to any of the tenants operating at the airport was 81 (69, 90) percent for small hub airports, 78 (76, 80) percent for non-hub airports, 44 (42, 47) percent for non-primary commercial service airports, and 16 (13, 19) percent for general aviation and reliever airports. The margins of error between the estimate for the small hub airports and the upper or lower bounds were greater than 10 percentage points. This estimate should be interpreted with caution.

[60] When asked to describe types of rent or other relief provided to tenants at the airport, 289 airports provided a valid written response. Of these responses, 152 airports stated they deferred payments for tenants, 117 stated they waived payments from tenants, and 77 airports stated they changed and/or adjusted leases and agreements, including reducing rates and fees. Airports may have reported taken more than one measure, so totals will not add up to 100 percent.

[61] As mentioned above, airlines and aviation manufacturers reported using the tax provisions in the CARES Act, including deferring employer payroll taxes, claiming employee retention credits, and carrying back five years net operating losses arising in tax years beginning in 2018, 2019, and 2020. These provisions were not limited to aviation industry businesses. Pub. L. No. 116-136, §§ 2301-2303, 134 Stat. at 347-56. The Consolidated Appropriations Act, 2021 made a number of changes to these provisions, including extending the availability of credits, among other changes. Pub. L. No. 116-260, div. N, §§ 206-207, 134 Stat. at 3059-65.

operating loss carryback provision that enabled it to record tax benefits of nearly $1.2 billion. The five manufacturers we spoke to did not pursue CARES Act loans. Generally, representatives told us they preferred maintaining flexibility in their business decision-making and chose not to pursue such loans because the requirements associated with accepting assistance—which included maintaining certain employment levels–were too restrictive.[62]

Some aviation businesses, including smaller companies in the manufacturing supply chain, received Paycheck Protection Program (PPP) loans to help sustain them through the period of decreased demand during the pandemic.[63] Representatives from one large manufacturer told us they understood that a number of the companies in their supply chain had received PPP loans, and that those loans

---

[62] Under the Section 4003 Loan Program, recipients agreed to maintain employment levels to the extent practicable and in any case not reduce employment levels by more than 10 percent until September 30, 2020. CARES Act, § 4003(c)(2)(G), 134 Stat. at 471. Under other programs, including PSP1, PSP2, and PSP3, recipients agreed to refrain from conducting involuntary furloughs. CARES Act, § 4114(a)(1), 134 Stat. at 499; Consolidated Appropriations Act, 2021, § 404, 134 Stat.at 2055; American Rescue Plan Act of 2021, § 7301, 135 Stat. at 104-05. Additionally, the American Rescue Plan Act of 2021, passed in March 2021, included $3 billion to establish an Aviation Manufacturing Jobs Protection program. Through this program, the Department of Transportation (DOT) is to provide up to $3 billion in funding to eligible manufacturing companies to pay up to half of their compensation costs for certain categories of employees, for up to sixmonths.

[63] The CARES Act and the Paycheck Protection Program and Health Care Enhancement Act appropriated a total of $670 billion for the Paycheck Protection Program (PPP) under the Small Business Administration's (SBA) 7(a) small business lending program. PPP loans are made at 1 percent interest and will be fully forgiven if certain conditions are met. These loans can be used for payroll and certain non-payroll costs. In general, small businesses with 500 or fewer employees, including tax-exempt nonprofit organizations, veterans organizations, and tribal businesses were eligible. Businesses in certain industries with more than 500 employees were eligible for loans. We previously reviewed the characteristics of PPP loans and the trends in small business and lender participation in PPP. See *Paycheck Protection Program: Program Changes Increased Lending to the Smallest Businesses and in Underserved Locations*, GAO-21-601 (Washington, D.C.: Sept. 21, 2021). We also reviewed aspects of SBA's implementation of the PPP, including safeguards that SBA put in place to prevent improper payments and fraud. See *Paycheck Protection Program: SBA Added Program Safeguards, but Additional Actions Are Needed,* GAO-21-577 (Washington, D.C.: July 29, 2021). Additionally, GAO previously found that SBA could take actions to improve oversight and fraud risk management of the PPP program. See, for example, *COVID-19 Loans: SBA has Begun to Take Steps to Improve Oversight and Fraud Risk Management*, GAO-21-498T (Washington, D.C.: Apr. 20, 2021); *Small Business Administration: Actions Needed to Improve COVID-19 Loans' Internal Controls and Reduce Their Susceptibility to Fraud*, GAO-21-472T (Washington, D.C.: Mar. 24, 2021); and *Small Business Administration: Steps Needed to Address COVID-19 Loan's Susceptibility to Fraud*, GAO-21-449T (Washington, D.C.: Mar. 25, 2021).

were a significant help for businesses that had been affected by the grounding of the Boeing 737 MAX aircraft in addition to the COVID-19 pandemic.

- *Repair station operators:* Treasury executed CARES Act loans totaling $19 million with five of the 41 repair station operators that applied to the program.[64] In addition to assistance from Treasury loans, the three rounds of PSP made up to $5 billion in financial assistance payments available to certain aviation contractors, including repair station operators. Two of the three repair station operators we interviewed received between $46 and $51 million in first-round PSP assistance payments. Representatives from one repair station operator said they used the assistance to retain their experienced workforce, perform necessary maintenance on their tooling and equipment, and perform training to keep their workforce current, among other things.
- *Cargo airlines:* Of the $4 billion appropriated for cargo airlines under the first round of PSP assistance to cover payroll expenses, only a fraction of the funding was used—thirty-nine cargo airlines received over $828 million in assistance.[65] Two cargo airlines received over two-thirds of these funds—$568 million. The two charter cargo airlines we spoke with received $35 million and $22 million of first-round PSP assistance. Representatives from both cargo airlines emphasized the importance of the support, stating that the assistance was critical in helping them through the first few months of the pandemic when they experienced a large decrease in demand. Representatives from one of the charter cargo airlines stated that without the PSP assistance, their airline would not have been in a financial position to survive the 3 to 4 months it took for their cargo business to return. They used the assistance to keep employees in place so that they were available when demand returned.

---

[64] In previous work we reported that representatives from smaller businesses told us the Treasury loan program did not work or did not work as well as it could have. See GAO-21-551.

[65] In October 2020, Representative James E. Clyburn, Chairman of the Select Subcommittee on the Coronavirus Crisis, sent letters to four cargo airlines that received a total of more than $630 million in PSP assistance, stating that it had appeared that the airlines "had financial success" during the COVID-19 pandemic. His letters called on the airlines to return the PSP assistance or demonstrate that they needed the funds to keep workers on their payroll, as Congress intended. As of September 2021, these airlines have not returned the funds. Assistance for cargo airlines was not included in the subsequent federal COVID-19 relief programs.

Aviation and Aerospace Stakeholders Raised Funding in the Financial Markets

In addition to receiving assistance from the various federal COVID-19 relief programs, many commercial aviation and aerospace stakeholders also raised funding in the financial markets to position themselves to maintain business viability until demand recovers. Representatives from several aviation industry associations and credit rating agencies told us that assistance from the CARES Act provided a degree of assurance in the stability of the market that enabled private lenders to invest in the aviation industry with greater confidence that they would be able to recoup their investments.

Major U.S. passenger airlines added an estimated $58 billion in private and federal long-term debt by the end of 2020, with their interest expenses expected to more than double in the next few years, according to A4A. As discussed earlier, throughout 2020, airlines were expending cash reserves at a rate faster than revenues could replenish and recognized that additional financing was needed to manage the dramatic drop in passenger revenue and cover fixed costs. According to public SEC financial reports, airlines issued or entered into new secured notes, loan facilities, and new aircraft financings, and raised cash proceeds from the issuance and sale of common stock, among other actions. For example, United Airlines reported $16 billion in proceeds from the issuance of debt and $2.1 billion in proceeds from equity issuance in 2020, with a total of $27.2 billion in debt and finance lease obligations at the end of 2020. Four passenger airlines—American Airlines, Hawaiian Airlines, Sun Country, and United Airlines—also turned to the financial markets in the first half of 2021 to raise funds that allowed them to pay back their CARES Act loans from the federal government.[66]

In some cases, aviation stakeholders pursued financing instead of federal COVID-19 relief assistance, citing various reasons they did not seek government financial support. Representatives from an aviation manufacturer described the provisions attached to the CARES Act loans as too restrictive and costly, stating that the company was not interested in providing the government with an equity stake or restricting its ability to reduce employment, as required by the loan program. Instead, representatives told us the manufacturer was able access the credit markets to obtain needed capital

[66] Two additional airlines—Alaska Airlines and SkyWest—also paid back their CARES Act loans from the federal government in the first half of 2021; however, their publicly available financial statements do not indicate the specific source of the funding used to repay these loans.

after the Federal Reserve's willingness to backstop the credit markets opened up credit options.[67] Separately, another manufacturer was able to issue $25 billion in new long-term debt in April 2020 to bolster its liquidity and thus did not pursue any CARES Act loans.

Aviation and Aerospace Stakeholders Took Steps to Mitigate the Spread of COVID-19

Protecting Employee Health

Stakeholders across aviation and aerospace sectors reported taking actions to protect employee health in 2020. These include such actions as requiring and providing masks, providing other personal protective equipment, implementing social distancing, and allowing employees to work from home when possible.[68] For example, representatives from a network airline reported providing on-site COVID-19 testing at its airport hubs and providing at-home testing for U.S. based employees.[69] Airlines also reported implementing remote work for employees able to do so, such as support center staff. Similarly, representatives from airports told us they implemented mask and social distancing requirements for employees and allowed some staff to work remotely.[70] Representatives from a cargo airline with its own repair station told us that to maintain social distancing among employees, they had to limit the number of mechanics working on a given aircraft as well as the number of

---

[67] We previously reported on the lending programs the Board of Governors of the Federal Reserve System authorized to ensure the flow of credit to various parts of the economy affected by the COVID-19 pandemic. See GAO, *Federal Reserve Lending Programs: Use of CARES Act-Supported Programs Has Been Limited and Flow of Credit Has Generally Improved,* GAO-21-180 (Washington, D.C.: Dec. 10, 2020).

[68] Personal protective equipment includes items such as N95 respirators, surgical and non-surgical masks, face shields and goggles, and gloves, among other items. Social distancing, also known as physical distancing, is the practice of maintaining physical distance from others and avoiding large gatherings, with the intent of reducing the rate of transmission of infectious diseases. COVID-19 brought social distancing practices to the forefront worldwide as a means of controlling local spread of the disease.

[69] Diagnostic testing for COVID-19 is critical to controlling and understanding the spread of the virus, according to the CDC. We previously reported on the types of COVID-19 testing in GAO, *Science & Tech Spotlight: COVID-19 Testing,* GAO-20-584SP (Washington, D.C.: May 20, 2020).

[70] Within commercial airports, the Transportation Security Administration (TSA) has responsibility for passenger screening checkpoints. For a review of measures implemented by TSA to protect its screening workforce and the traveling public, see GAO, *COVID-19: TSA Could Better Monitor Its Efforts to Reduce Infectious Disease Spread at Checkpoints*, GAO-21-364 (Washington, D.C.: June 14, 2021).

mechanics working on the same part of an aircraft at the same time. Representatives from manufacturers told us they implemented temperature checks and added social distancing where possible, including in production areas.[71] Representatives from two manufacturers also told us they developed protocols for contact tracing if employees reported positive COVID-19 infections.[72]

Protecting Passengers and Increasing Confidence in the Air Travel Experience

Airlines and airports also took actions in 2020 with an intent to protect passengers and increase passenger confidence in the air travel experience.[73] Representatives from airlines and airports we spoke to emphasized the enhanced cleaning protocols they implemented throughout their airports and on aircraft. Some airlines also changed their onboard food and beverage services to reduce interactions between passengers and crew and blocked the sale of middle seats to allow for greater distancing between passengers. Representatives from one airline and seven airports also told us they implemented contactless technology to reduce interaction between passengers and employees, such as adding automated bag drops and biometric ID checks. Representatives from six airports also told us it was important to implement consistent messaging and expectation setting about mask and social distancing requirements throughout their airports to help passengers navigate differences in requirements at different destinations (see Figure 5). While some of these measures, such as contactless technology, may be maintained in the long-term, others have been changing as public health needs have evolved with the rollout of vaccines and the beginning of pandemic recovery.[74]

---

[71] Centers for Disease Control and Prevention (CDC) guidance states that screening employees for symptoms of COVID-19, such as a fever, is an optional strategy employers may use to reduce the spread of COVID-19 in the workplace.

[72] Contact tracing is a process in which public health officials attempt to limit disease transmission by identifying infected individuals, notifying their "contacts"—all the people they may have transmitted the disease to—and asking infected individuals and their contacts to quarantine, if appropriate.

[73] We have not evaluated the effectiveness of these actions, but we are currently reviewing the research surrounding the transmission of communicable disease in air travel.

[74] Two COVID-19 vaccines using a two-dose regimen (Pfizer and Moderna) were authorized for emergency use in December 2020 and a third, one-dose vaccine (Johnson & Johnson) was authorized in February 2021. As of June 23, 2021, about 323 million vaccine doses have been administered, according to data reported to CDC, and about 53.1 percent of the U.S. population 12 and over—almost 150.7 million individuals—have been fully vaccinated. For additional information, see GAO-21-551.

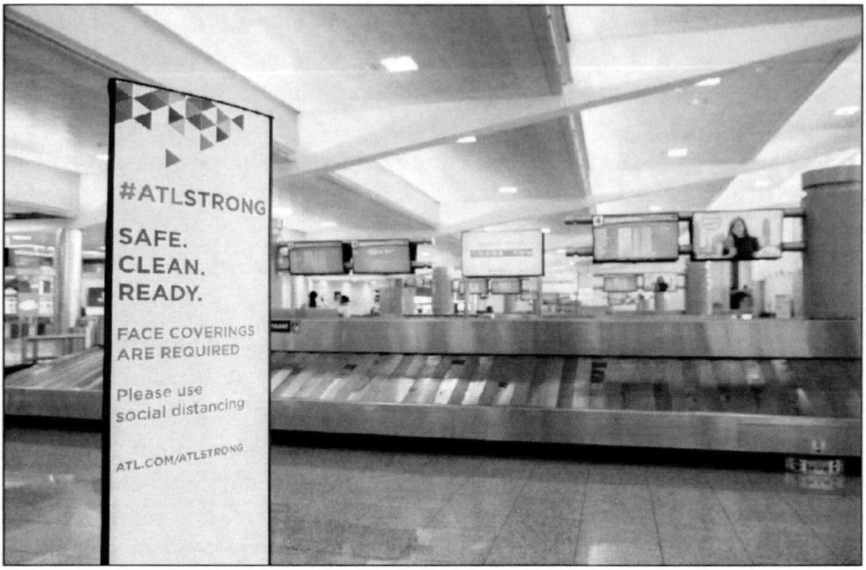
#ATLSTRONG
SAFE.
CLEAN.
READY.
FACE COVERINGS
ARE REQUIRED
Please use
social distancing
ATL.COM/ATLSTRONG

Source: Hartsfield-Jackson Atlanta International Airport; © Decisive Moment Photojournalism. | GAO-22-104429.

Figure 5. Sign at Hartsfield-Jackson Atlanta International Airport with COVID-19 Requirements and Reminders.

FAA Provided Airlines and Other Aviation Sectors Temporary Relief from Some Regulatory Requirements and Selected Stakeholders Said the Changes Were Helpful

FAA Granted Airlines' Requests for Temporary Relief from Meeting Certain Regulatory Requirements

In March 2020, FAA began granting specific and temporary regulatory relief, including granting regulatory waivers, approving operational adjustments, and issuing guidance, in response to requests from airlines, airports, and their industry associations (see Table 1). As aviation activity declined with the start of the pandemic, airlines and aviation associations sought FAA's assistance to ease regulatory and operational requirements that they claimed negatively affected the safety and continuity of aviation operations. For example, Airlines for America and National Air Transportation Association petitioned FAA on behalf of their members for exemptions to regulations requiring crewmembers to don emergency equipment (e.g., oxygen masks and life vests) during training.[75] These associations explained that, without a temporary exemption, such procedures could lead to the transmission of COVID-19. Associations also petitioned FAA for regulatory relief that would allow them to make operational changes. For example, Airlines for America petitioned FAA for exemptions that would allow airlines to transport cargo in a plane's passenger cabin when no passengers were present.[76] Airlines for America explained that some airlines might want to use their excess capacity to carry cargo, including critical medical cargo.

During 2020, FAA granted stakeholders' requests for extensions of regulatory relief as it determined that pandemic conditions warranted relief, but as of July 2021, most of FAA's relief measures had expired. By mid-2021, the public health emergency diminished, aviation operations began to normalize, and aviation stakeholders did not petition FAA for further extensions. In granting some extensions, FAA identified additional ways to mitigate potential safety impacts that might result from the extensions. For example, FAA phased out medical certification grace periods for crewmembers who had already been granted extensions and extended the grace period relief to new cohorts of crewmembers facing imminent expiration dates.

Table 1. Federal Aviation Administration (FAA) pandemic relief actions, March 2020-July 2021

FAA Relief Actions (as of July 2021)	Effective Date/Expiration Date (if applicable)
Regulatory Relief	
FAA's exemptions—Exemption 18510 and 18511—extended the timeframes for charter carriers' and commercial airlines ground personnel, crewmembers, and dispatchers to complete recurring training and qualification requirements. FAA granted 3 extensions for each exemption. See Regulatory Docket No. FAA-2020-0292 and FAA-2020-0308 respectively.	March 2020/ March 2021
FAA's exemptions—Exemption 18515 and 18516—extended the duration of medical certificates for pilots and flight engineers operating flights outside of the U.S. FAA subsequently broadened the medical relief to all pilots and flight engineers through the issuance of the Special Federal Aviation Regulation (see below). See Regulatory Docket No. FAA-2020-0317 and FAA-2020-0318 respectively.	March 2020/ June 2020

[75] 14 C.F.R. § 121.417. See Regulatory Docket No. FAA-2020-0307 and FAA-2020-0291.
[76] See Regulatory Docket No. FAA-2020-0492.

Table 1. Continued

FAA Relief Actions (as of July 2021)	Effective Date/Expiration Date (if applicable)
Regulatory Relief	
FAA's exemptions—Exemption 18509 and 18512—allowed airline crewmembers to use alternate means when conducting required emergency procedures during training, testing, and checking. For example, crewmembers were exempted from having to don oxygen masks or life vests during training. FAA granted 3 extensions for each exemption. See Regulatory Docket No. FAA-2020-0291 and FAA-2020-0307 respectively.	March 2020/ March 2021
FAA waived the minimum usage requirement for airlines using runway slots (i.e., a take-off or landing) associated with a scheduled nonstop flight between John F. Kennedy International, New York LaGuardia, and Ronald Reagan Washington National airports and other points that were cancelled as a result of pandemic-related impacts.	March 2020/ October 2021
FAA also provided similar relief to airlines using Chicago O'Hare International, Newark Liberty International, Los Angeles International, and San Francisco International airports that prioritized flights cancelled due to pandemic-related impacts for purposes of establishing an airline's operational baseline in the next corresponding season. FAA granted 3 extensions. See Notice of Limited Waiver of the Slot Usage Requirement 85 Fed. Reg. 15,018 (Mar. 16, 2020).[a]	
FAA's partial exemptions—Exemption 18561 and 18584—allowed commercial airlines to carry cargo on seats and floors in airplanes when no passengers are transported. FAA granted 2 extensions for exemption 18561 and 1 extension for exemption 18584. See Regulatory Docket No. FAA-2020-0429.	May 2020/July 2021
FAA's exemption—Exemption 18522—allowed flight attendants to relocate seats they would normally occupy in order to comply with recommendations from the Centers for Disease Control and Prevention concerning proximity to others. It also waived the requirement to don oxygen masks and other equipment during passenger safety briefings. FAA granted 3 extensions. See Regulatory Docket No. FAA-2020-0372.	April 2020/June 2021
FAA's Special Federal Aviation Regulation 118 (SFAR) provided relief to training, testing, qualification, and medical certification requirements pertaining to pilots, mechanics, and dispatchers. This included granting relief for non-commercial operations to individuals or companies that were unable to meet training duration and renewal requirements. The relief allowed the continued use of pilots and other crewmembers in support of essential operations. The SFAR also made it easier for operators to move aircraft from one storage facility to another. FAA granted 2 extensions. Relief from Certain Persons and Operations During the Coronavirus Disease 2019 (COVID-19) Outbreak, 85 Fed. Reg. 26,326 (May 4, 2020).	April 2020/ April 2021

FAA Relief Actions (as of July 2021)	Effective Date/Expiration Date (if applicable)
Regulatory Relief	
FAA's exemption—Exemption 18537—extended the timeframes for air ambulance personnel to complete recurring training and testing requirements. FAA granted 2 extensions. See Regulatory Docket No. FAA-2020-0412.	April 2020/ December 2020
Operational Adjustments	
FAA allowed airlines to park unused aircraft that overflowed ordinary parking areas at airports and issued guidance to airport operators on developing a plan to park overflow aircraft and when to close runways and taxiways for temporary aircraft parking.	March 2020/Dates varied but most overflow aircraft removed by late fall 2020
FAA reduced operating hours of some air traffic control towers in response to decreased air traffic operations.	April 2020/ March 2021
FAA allowed airlines that temporarily removed aircraft from service to deviate from their normal aircraft maintenance program while the aircraft was grounded.	June 2020/ August 2021
Operational Adjustments	
FAA closed air traffic control towers during COVID-19 outbreaks.	July 2020/Ongoing
Guidance and Enforcement Actions	
The Department of Transportation (DOT) issued an enforcement notice to international passengers that airlines may refuse transportation to passengers with COVID-19 symptoms because they pose a direct health and safety threat.	March 2020
DOT issued an enforcement notice to airlines requiring prompt refunds for cancelled flights.	April 2020
FAA issued health and safety alerts and policies covering a range of topics from health guidance for crews to prevent spread of COVID-19, to safely transporting dry ice, to the observation period after pilots and air traffic controllers get vaccinated.	Various
FAA/DOT, in collaboration with Department of Homeland Security and Department of Health and Human Services, issued an update to Runway to Recovery, a guide for airlines and airports to mitigate the public health risks of COVID-19. FAA/DOT published an update in December 2020.	July 2020
FAA directed its investigative personnel to take stricter action in the form of civil penalties against unruly airline passengers who assault, threaten, intimidate, or interfere with airline crew members.	January 2021

Source: GAO analysis of Federal Aviation Administration information. | GAO-22-104429.

[a]See also Notice of Extension of Limited Waiver of the Minimum Slot Usage Requirement, 85 Fed. Reg. 21,500 (Apr. 17, 2020); Extension of Limited Waiver of the Minimum Slot Usage Requirement, 85 Fed. Reg. 63,335 (Oct. 7, 2020); and FAA Policy Statement: Limited, Conditional Extension of COVID-19 Related Relief for the Summer 2021 Scheduling Season (Docket No. FAA-202-0862) (Jan. 13, 2021).

According to FAA officials, the agency granted regulatory relief and issued guidance using its standard processes in most cases. For example, FAA followed its standard procedure in publicizing airlines' petitions for regulatory exemption and accepting public comments on those petitions.[77] However, FAA expedited some processes, which, according to FAA officials, helped both the airlines and FAA. For example, FAA did not require airlines to submit petitions for exemption 120 days before the desired effective date of the exemption,[78] allowed industry associations to submit petitions on behalf of their members, and granted exemptions to all affected airlines that submitted a letter of intent.[79] This change expedited relief because it removed the requirement that each airline must petition individually for an exemption and thus removed the need for FAA to evaluate multiple individual petitions for the same relief. FAA's exemption letters, waivers, and Special Federal Aviation Regulation (SFAR)[80] summarize the agency's reasons for granting relief, its assessment of potential safety impacts, and any additional requirements airlines accepting relief must follow.

According to FAA officials, FAA's foremost considerations in evaluating the stakeholder requests for regulatory relief were whether the relief measure would have an adverse effect on safety or would not be in the public interest, and would facilitate the continuity of aviation operations.

---

[77] FAA published some petitions for regulatory exemptions in a regulatory docket and other petitions in the *Federal Register* depending on the waiver sought. For example, in one regulatory exemption, FAA found good cause under 14 C.F.R. § 11.87 not to publish a summary of the petition in the *Federal Register* because "delaying action on the petition would have an adverse and potentially immediate impact on the petitioner's ability to ensure continuity of critical air ambulance operations essential to the public interest." In the Matter of the Petition of Air Medical Operators Association, Exemption No. 18537 (Apr. 30, 2020).

[78] Aviation stakeholders affected by a regulation in Title 14 of the Code of Federal Regulations may petition for an exemption from any rule issued by FAA under its statutory authority. The regulations governing this process (14 C.F.R. pt. 11) describe the steps for petitioning for exemptions. These steps include submitting the petition 120 days before it is needed to take effect, describing the relief needed, reasons it would not affect safety, and other information. FAA publishes information about petitions for exemption in the *Federal Register*. 14 C.F.R. § 11.85.

[79] FAA directed airlines that were requesting an exemption to submit a letter of intent to FAA. The letter of intent required the airline to affirm its request to use the exemption and its intentions to comply with the conditions and limitation of the exemption. Some exemptions contained other requirements, such as evaluating and describing how the airline would prevent negative safety impacts.

[80] According to FAA, an SFAR pertaining to airspace is typically a temporary rule to address a temporary situation. Further, FAA notes that an SFAR is generally not used to replace or enforce regulations that are to remain in effect for many years. Consequently, an SFAR has an expiration date, usually no more than 3 years from its effective date. SFARs are listed at the beginning of the most relevant Code of Federal Regulations, and may be cross-referenced to other regulations. SFARs can prohibit, restrict, or impose additional requirements to operate in the airspace to which the SFAR applies.

FAA officials said that focusing on aviation stakeholder requests enabled the agency to quickly address the most critical operational issues.

FAA took other actions in addition to providing regulatory relief. For example, in March 2020, FAA created a rapid response team that was a focal point for gathering and responding to airport operators' and other stakeholders' questions and concerns. According to FAA officials, the team's main purpose was to create a channel of communication with industry, quickly tackle any issue brought to its attention, and elevate issues that need broader attention. For example, the team fielded questions ranging from where to obtain hand sanitizer to who needs to know about overflow aircraft parking plans. Since its inception, the team has cataloged over 750 requests for information and policy decisions.

Airlines Credited FAA for Quick Actions in Support of Continuing Operations

The airlines we contacted commented that FAA's actions demonstrated its ability to provide operational relief quickly. FAA officials stated that the agency's efficiency was due in part to industry input because industry stakeholders—particularly airline associations—identified regulatory relief that was critical to continuing operations. According to FAA officials, some exemptions were beneficial to airlines and the public because the exemptions enabled airlines to maintain qualified crewmembers. These officials said other exemptions were beneficial because they reduced crewmembers' potential exposure to COVID-19 during training or operations and two airlines we contacted agreed. For example, one airline said that by allowing flight attendants to sit in seats throughout the plane at a distance from crewmembers and passengers (not in their designated jump seat), FAA likely helped airlines reduce the spread of the virus. FAA officials stated that it was up to each airline whether to apply for regulatory relief and that not all airlines did so. The airlines we contacted said they chose the exemptions that fit their operations. One airline ceased training pilots on aircraft used for international flights while another allowed its flight dispatchers to work from home. One airline official stated that although exempting crewmembers from demonstrating safety equipment was likely only marginally helpful, pilots and flight attendants appreciated that their safety was being acknowledged.

The Extent of Industry Recovery Remains Uncertain and Stakeholders Identified Considerations for Potential Federal Support

Uncertainty About the Ongoing Recovery Remains Despite Rebound in U.S. Leisure Travel

Recovery in U.S. Leisure Travel Is Slowing

Passenger airlines experienced a resurgence in demand for domestic leisure travel in the spring and summer of 2021; however, their recovery has been slowed by operational challenges and concerns about the COVID-19 Delta variant. In March 2021, the credit rating agency Fitch Ratings noted that a decline in COVID-19 death rates could be sufficient to loosen pandemic restrictions, increase consumer comfort with the idea of traveling, and begin a rebound in air travel.[81] Fitch cautioned that the emergence of highly transmissible variants could extend the pandemic and delay a recovery in air travel in the United States and Canada.

According to the most recent BTS data available as of September 2021, passenger airlines carried 66 million passengers within the United States in July 2021, which was more than double passenger levels in either January or February 2021, and a roughly 191 percent increase compared to July 2020. In response to increasing demand for domestic leisure travel, U.S. airlines began adapting flight operations and their workforce levels in spring 2021. For example, in April 2021, United Airlines announced plans to hire 300 new pilots, and American Airlines announced it would add 150 new routes on its network in summer 2021.

On June 11, 2021, 2 million people crossed TSA airport security checkpoints, the highest level since March 7, 2020.[82]

However, in certain cases, the fast rebound in demand for air travel has exceeded airlines' ability to return capacity to service, resulting in cancelled and rescheduled flights. For example, Spirit Airlines cancelled more than

---

[81] Fitch Ratings, *North American Airline and Airport Pressures to Ease, Accelerating Recovery Later This Year*, Fitch Wire (Mar., 11, 2021).

[82] In June, the Centers for Disease Control and Prevention (CDC) updated its guidance to advise that fully vaccinated travelers could safely travel within the United States and U.S. territories provided that they continue to wear a mask as required on planes, buses, trains, and other forms of public transportation traveling into, within, or out of the United States and while indoors at U.S. transportation hubs such as airports and stations. The CDC also advised that travelers follow all state and local recommendations and requirements, including for mask wearing and social distancing.

2,000 flights between late July and early August. According to airlines, the increase in cancellations are due to a combination of staffing shortages, weather, and information technology problems.[83] As noted above, many airlines reduced their staffing through voluntary and involuntary measures as a cost cutting measure and are now trying to hire and train more staff. However, retraining and recertifying some staff, especially pilots, can be a lengthy process.

The emergence and spread of the COVID-19 Delta variant appears to have contributed to weakened demand for air travel in late summer 2021. On July 27, 2021, prompted by a rise in COVID-19 case and hospitalization rates around the country, the CDC released updated guidance urging an increase in vaccination coverage around the country and recommending that people in areas of substantial or high transmission wear a mask in public or indoor places, even if they are fully vaccinated. On August 11, Southwest Airlines reported that bookings have slowed and trip cancellations have increased, which the airline attributed to the recent rise in COVID-19 cases associated with the Delta variant. According to the Airlines Reporting Corporation, tickets sales for the week of August 9 were down 41 percent compared to 2019, the worst differential between 2021 and 2019 sales since mid-May. The TSA reported that it screened 1,607,238 air passengers on August 17, a 28 percent decline from the 2,238,462 passengers screened on August 1. However, this decline also coincided with the summer travel season winding down; in August 2019, there was a 16 percent decline in passengers screened over the same period.

International and Business Air Travel Continue to Lag

Although U.S. airlines experienced a rebound in demand for domestic leisure travel in 2021, demand for international and business travel has lagged and is likely to continue to do so, according to aviation industry stakeholders including credit rating agencies and consulting firms. As discussed previously, international and business travel are critical contributors to the profitability of network airlines. According to McKinsey, for example, business travelers can account for 55–75 percent of airline profits.[84] Some stakeholders project that it will take until sometime in the 2023–2025 period for a return to pre-

[83] In 2019, we reported on airline technology issues, noting that federal regulators do not have data on airline technology outages, but we noted at least 34 instances of outages and the vast majority resulted in delays and cancellations. GAO, *Commercial Aviation: Information on Airline IT Outages*, GAO-19-514 (Washington DC; Jun 12, 2019).

[84] McKinsey & Company, *For corporate travel, a long recovery ahead* (August 2020).

pandemic traffic levels. These stakeholders note that international and business travel recovery are also dependent on factors including the progress of vaccine dissemination outside of the U.S. and the extent to which businesses continue to use videoconferencing in lieu of in-person meetings.

Demand for international air travel remains depressed in late summer 2021, and may not recover to pre-pandemic levels for several years, according to industry observers. International air travel remains roughly 40 percent below 2019 levels in early September 2021, according to A4A, and the consulting firm Oliver Wyman has projected that, based on pandemic-related travel restrictions, the growing number of infections due to COVID-19 variants, and the lack of progress in vaccine dissemination outside of the United States, international travel will not recover until 2023 or 2024.[85]

Industry analysts also expect a lag in the return of demand for business air travel. Moody's reported in March 2021 that the extent to which virtual meetings will replace business travel in the longer term is unknown, and estimated that 10–30 percent of this segment may not return after the pandemic. According to Moody's, factors that may limit the recovery of business travel include (1) greater use and familiarity with virtual meeting technologies, (2) a desire to continue to reap savings from reduced travel that were gained during the pandemic, (3) an increased interest in reducing carbon emissions, and (4) a greater emphasis on prioritizing travel dollars where they provide the greatest benefit, such as when it helps to promote customer relationships or revenue generation. Notably, Moody's reported that while travel to meet with customers may return relatively quickly, trips related to conventions or trade shows could be slower to recover. Forecasts from several industry observers vary, but generally converge on expecting a multi-year period for a return to pre- pandemic levels of business travel. For example, Moody's forecasted in March 2021 that business travel will not reach 2019 levels until at least 2024,[86] and McKinsey estimated in April 2021 that business travel will likely recover to 80 percent of pre-pandemic levels by 2024.[87] The U.S. Travel Association and research firm Tourism Economics forecast in July 2021 that business travel will return to 76 percent of 2019 levels in 2022, 92 percent in 2023, and finally exceed 2019 levels in 2024.

---

[85] Oliver Wyman, *Airline Economic Analysis 2020-21.*

[86] Moody's Investors Service, *Business Travel Faces Higher Substitution Risk Post- COVID, But Airlines Will Adapt* (Mar. 24, 2021).

[87] McKinsey & Company, *Back to the future? Airline sector poised for change post-COVID- 19* (April 2021).

The Aviation Industry's Recovery to Financial Health Depends on How It Adapts to the Evolving Market in the Coming Years

The recovery of the aviation industry to profitability and financial health depends on how various aviation sectors—predominantly airlines, but also airports, manufacturers, and repair station operators—are able to adapt to evolving market conditions in the coming years. How sectors adapt, in turn, may result in changes to business models and operations.

Passenger Airlines

Industry analysts suggest that based on the expected lag in recovery for international and business air travel, airlines that serve primarily domestic routes and rely on leisure travel, such as low-cost airlines, are better positioned for near-term recovery than airlines that have focused on business and international travel. For example, Delta Air Lines, United Airlines, and American Airlines generate at least a third of their revenue from business travelers, according to Moody's.[88] As a result, these airlines may face challenges in regaining their previous level of profitability if demand for business travel does not quickly return to pre- pandemic levels. Airlines may act to offset the possible effects of a slow recovery in business travel by more conservatively managing capacity dedicated to such routes, increasing their focus on leisure travel, and raising leisure fares, according to Moody's. In particular, they may choose to reconfigure aircraft cabins to focus on serving more leisure travelers, with less business-class seating and more economy or premium seating. According to Oliver Wyman's *Airline Economic Analysis 2020–2021*, a near-term focus on leisure travel will alter aspects of airlines' demand forecasting and capacity planning, as patterns of leisure demand are different than business demand.

Airports

U.S. airport operators are also likely to face several challenges resulting from reduced air travel demand caused by the pandemic. In a dynamic similar to that facing U.S. airlines, airports oriented toward domestic leisure travel are expected to rebound more quickly than international gateway airports or those with a high reliance on business travelers, according to a March 2021 Fitch Ratings report. In January 2021, S&P Global Ratings reported that airports that have traditionally relied on strong business and international travel may

[88] Moody's Investors Service, *Business Travel Faces Higher Substitution Risk Post- COVID, But Airlines Will Adapt* (Mar. 24, 2021).

have more difficulty or take longer to compensate for a loss of non-aeronautical revenues from parking, concessions, and rental car operations if the travelers that patronize these businesses are slow to return.[89]

Airports may also face challenges in capital planning moving forward, as airports reported deferring or delaying such projects during the pandemic. According to Airports Council International–North America, airports face a backlog of $115 billion in planned capital investments. Among other capital planning considerations, some smaller airports may face challenges in accommodating increasing passenger volumes with social distancing protocols still in place. For example, one industry analyst told us that airports that are near outdoor leisure destinations like national parks are experiencing increased demand, but have comparatively small physical footprints.

Manufacturers and Repair Station Operators

Evolving market conditions are affecting the airline industry's demand for new aircraft as well as for maintenance services, with associated effects for manufacturers, repair stations, and other businesses in the aviation supply chain.

- *Manufacturing.* According to S&P Global Ratings, Airbus and Boeing reduced production of most aircraft models by 30–50 percent in 2020 in response to airline decisions to defer or cancel new aircraft orders. S&P forecasts that aircraft production rates are likely to remain at this level in 2021 and may not reach 2018 levels until 2024.[90] Based on recovering demand for domestic leisure travel, airline demand for narrowbody aircraft will likely recover before demand for the widebodies used for long-haul, international travel.[91] Boeing, for example, reported slowing production of the widebody 787 aircraft from 14 per month before the pandemic to five per month as of March 31, 2021 based on reduced customer demand. However, according to Boeing's data on airplane gross orders, orders for aircraft have increased recently. In January and February 2021, Boeing received orders for 86 aircraft; from March through July, the manufacturer received orders for 544 aircraft, the bulk of which are for the narrowbody 737 MAX.

---

[89] S&P Global Ratings, *Outlook for U.S. Not-for-Profit Transportation Infrastructure: Light at Tunnel's End–But How Long is the Tunnel?* (Jan. 13, 2021).

[90] S&P Global Ratings, *Industry Top Trends 2021–Aerospace and Defense* (Dec. 10, 2020).

[91] Narrowbody aircraft have one aisle, whereas widebody aircraft have two aisles.

- *Maintenance, Repair, and Overhaul.* A December 2020 report from S&P Global Ratings forecasted that repair stations may recover in line with increased demand for air travel as airlines bring aircraft back into service. Similarly, officials from the Aeronautical Repair Station Association (ARSA) told us in May 2021 that they are seeing a return in demand for aircraft maintenance service as network airlines return aircraft to service. According to ARSA, as demand has increased, pre-pandemic concerns about an industry shortage in aviation maintenance technicians have resumed.

Aviation Industry Stakeholders Identified Considerations for Potential Federal Support

During our review, aviation industry stakeholders identified several areas of concern for policymakers to consider as they determine how or whether to continue to assist the aviation industry as COVID-19 relief funds are expended and market conditions evolve. Additionally, stakeholders noted considerations for policymakers in preparing a federal aviation response to future pandemics.

Strengthening the Aviation Workforce Pipeline

As a result of workforce reductions undertaken in response to the pandemic, a key concern moving forward will be maintaining healthy workforce pipelines for key aviation professions including airline pilots and aviation maintenance technicians, according to representatives from airlines and repair stations we spoke with. These pipelines include collegiate training programs and apprenticeships. We have previously reported on industry concerns that an insufficient supply of airline pilots and maintenance technicians could develop as a result of retirements, education and training costs, and difficulty hiring individuals with desired experience levels.[92] An Oliver Wyman study forecasts that a pilot shortage—a concern before the pandemic—will reemerge quickly and may exceed 12,000 pilots by 2023.[93] Although reduced demand from the pandemic temporarily alleviated these pressures, they appear to have reemerged as firms face difficulty in replacing skilled aviation workers who

---

[92] GAO, *Aviation Workforce: Current and Future Availability of Airline Pilots*, GAO-14-232 (Washington, D.C.: Feb. 28, 2014), and *Aviation Workforce: Current and Future Availability of Aviation Maintenance and Engineering Professionals*, GAO-14-237 (Washington, D.C.: Feb. 28, 2014).

[93] Oliver Wyman, "After COVID-19, Aviation Faces a Pilot Shortage." March 2021.

were encouraged to retire, were laid off, or migrated to other industries during the industry downturn in 2020. In March 2021, the American Rescue Plan Act of 2021 was enacted, establishing the Aviation Manufacturing Jobs Protection (AMJP) Program. Through this program, DOT is to provide up to $3 billion in funding to eligible aviation manufacturing companies to pay up to half of their compensation costs for certain categories of employees, for up to six months.[94] As we testified in March 2021, aviation workforce retraining and efforts to strengthen the pipeline of new applicants for aviation careers, such as through apprenticeships and pathway programs, could help ensure the workforce is ready to respond to future air travel demand.[95]

Providing Small Communities Access to the National Transportation System

While communities of all sizes seek access to air service as a driver for attracting investment, generating employment, and providing mobility for citizens, as we have reported, small communities were collectively losing air service prior to COVID-19, and the pandemic may exacerbate this trend.[96] DOT has required airlines receiving payroll payments and loans to maintain some service levels to small communities, as authorized by COVID-19 relief laws. In addition, the Consolidated Appropriations Act, 2021 set aside up to $5 million of the $2 billion appropriated for Grants-in-Aid for Airports for the Small Community Air Service Development Program (SCASDP).[97] In addition, the Act directed that in allocating this funding and SCASDP funding for fiscal years 2019, 2020, and 2021, DOT give priority to communities that have had airline service reduced or suspended as a result of the pandemic.

As DOT ends these air service obligations in March 2022, some small communities may face a reduction in or a complete loss of air service as airlines focus on more profitable markets during recovery. Aviation stakeholders such as the Regional Airline Association have suggested that Congress address service reductions stemming from the pandemic by providing funding for Essential Air Service (EAS) and SCASDP to maintain

---

[94] § 7202, 135 Stat. 4, 103-04.

[95] GAO, *COVID-19 Pandemic: Preliminary Observations on Efforts toward and Factors Affecting the Aviation Industry's Recovery*, GAO-21-412T (Washington, D.C.: Mar. 2, 2021).

[96] GAO, *Small Community Air Service Development: Process for Awarding Grants Could Be Improved*, GAO-19-172 (Washington, D.C.: March 26, 2019), and *Commercial Aviation: Status of Air Service to Small Communities and the Federal Programs Involved*, GAO-14-454T (Washington, D.C.: April 30, 2014).

[97] SCASDP is a grant program designed to help small communities address air service and airfare issues. For more information, see GAO-19-172.

service to small communities.[98] We and others have found that a broader set of issues is driving the longer-term decline of air service to small communities, and solutions provided through other options such as bus service or unscheduled air taxi service, or in the longer term, Advanced Air Mobility technologies, may be worth consideration.[99]

Considering Future Financial Assistance

The airline industry received substantial financial support from several COVID-19 relief assistance programs that aided businesses and protected jobs, but some analysts noted potential downsides to that support. While this assistance helped businesses respond to the unprecedented demand shock by keeping many workers on the payroll and enabled airlines and other businesses to be better prepared to meet demand when it returned, some analysts believe that it also may have deterred market adjustments that likely would have occurred in the absence of substantial assistance.[100] For example, economic contraction and expansion—leading in some cases to mergers, restructuring, and liquidation—have been a feature of the airline industry since its deregulation in 1978. Despite the dramatic downturn in traffic and revenues, only two small airlines filed for bankruptcy in 2020.[101] Although it may be too soon to examine these issues empirically, some analysts believe that pandemic relief could have delayed industry adjustments that might have proven to be beneficial in the long run. For example, business failure and new entry can spur relatively rapid and substantive readjustments in business models at minimal cost to taxpayers. According to some analysts, financial support also rewarded management, creditors, and shareholders that were shielded from the

[98] The Airline Deregulation Act of 1978, which established the EAS program, specifies that if DOT determines that if air service will not be provided without subsidy, DOT shall use EAS program funds to award a subsidy to an airline willing to provide service. For more information, see GAO, *Commercial Aviation: Effects of Changes to the Essential Air Service Program, and Stakeholders' Views on Benefits, Challenges, and Potential Reforms*, GAO-20-74 (Washington, D.C.: Dec. 10, 2019).

[99] Department of Transportation, *Report of the Working Group on Improving Air Service to Small Communities* (Washington, D.C.: May 9, 2017), and GAO, *National Transportation System: Options and Analytical Tools to Strengthen DOT's Approach to Supporting Communities' Access to the System* (Washington, D.C.: July 17, 2009). See also The National Academies of Sciences, Engineering, and Medicine, *Advancing Aerial Mobility: A National Blueprint*, (Washington, D.C.: 2020).

[100] Veronique de Rugy and Gary Leff, *The Case Against Bailing Out the Airline Industry*, George Mason University Mercatus Center, March 2020.

[101] Ravn Air and Air Miami International filed for Chapter 11 bankruptcy in 2020.

financial consequences of risks they had assumed.[102] Additionally, analysts note that the industry might suffer if, based on the recent pandemic relief, airlines expect federal financial assistance when shocks to air travel demand occur in the future.[103] That expectation might limit the steps firms would otherwise take to prepare for future disruptions, and as such, could hamper the industry's development of longer-run resilience to respond to such events.

Preparing for the Next Pandemic

Several aviation stakeholders we spoke with in 2020 and early 2021, including representatives from airports and airlines, told us that passenger confidence in the air travel experience could have been restored more quickly if the federal government had provided greater coordination and guidance earlier in the pandemic regarding, among other things, COVID-19 testing, masking requirements, and baseline actions—such as sanitizing and updating signage—that airports and airlines could take.[104] For example, representatives from one airport told us that inconsistent passenger procedures between origin and destination airports were a major challenge, and that the federal government has a pivotal role to play in restoring passenger confidence in flying. Such federal coordination and guidance is consistent with our June 2020 matter urging Congress to take legislative action to require DOT to work with relevant agencies and stakeholders, such as the Department of Health and Human Services (HHS) and the Department of Homeland Security (DHS), to develop a national aviation preparedness plan for communicable disease outbreaks.[105] This plan would provide a mechanism for public health and

---

[102] Veronique de Rugy and Gary Leff, *The Case Against Bailing Out the Airline Industry*, George Mason University Mercatus Center, March 2020. See also Veronique de Rugy and Gary Leff, *The Economic Case Against a Second Airline Payroll Bailout*, George Mason University Mercatus Center, October 2020, and Hubert Horan, "The AirlineIndustry after COVID-19: Value Extraction or Recovery?" *American Affairs*, Spring 2021.

[103] Veronique de Rugy and Gary Leff, *The Case Against Bailing Out the Airline Industry*, George Mason University Mercatus Center, March 2020.

[104] These interviews were conducted before President Biden's January 2021 executive order requiring mask-wearing on certain domestic modes of transportation.

[105] In 2015, we recommended that the Secretary of Transportation work with relevant stakeholders, such as the Department of Health and Human Services (HHS), to develop a national aviation-preparedness plan for communicable diseases. DOT agreed that an aviation-preparedness plan is needed. DOT, however, maintains that those agencies that have both legal authority and expertise for emergency response and public health— namely the Department of Homeland Security (DHS) and HHS—are best positioned to take the lead role in developing such a plan. We continue to believe that DOT would be in the best position to lead the effort because FAA and DOT have stronger and deeper ties to, as well as oversight responsibility for, the relevant stakeholders that would be most involved in such a broad effort, namely airlines, airports, and other aviation stakeholders. In June 2020, we urged Congress to

aviation sectors to coordinate to limit the spread of communicable disease threats and minimize trade and travel impacts. Without such a plan, the U.S. may not be as prepared to minimize and quickly respond to future communicable disease threats. Members of the House and Senate have introduced bills in support of this matter. In February 2021, H.R. 884, the National Aviation Preparedness Plan Act of 2021,[106] was introduced in the House of Representatives, and in May 2021, the Ensuring Health Safety in the Skies Act of 2021,[107] was reported favorably out of the Senate Committee on Commerce, Science, and Transportation.

Agency Comments

We provided a copy of this report to DOT for review and comment. DOT provided technical comments, which we incorporated as appropriate.

We are sending copies of this report to the appropriate congressional committees, the Secretary of Transportation, and other interested parties. In addition, the report is available at no charge on the GAO website at http://www.gao.gov.

If you or your staff have any questions about this report, please contact Heather Krause at (202) 512-2834 or krauseh@gao.gov. Contact points for our Offices of Congressional Relations and Public Affairs may be found on the last page of this report. GAO staff who made key contributions to this report are listed in appendix III.

Heather Krause
Director, Physical Infrastructure Issues

take legislative action to require DOT to develop a national aviation-preparedness plan. See GAO-20-625.

[106] H.R. 884, 117th Cong. (2021).

[107] S. 82, 117th Cong. (2021).

List of Addressees

The Honorable Patrick Leahy
Chair
The Honorable Richard Shelby
Vice Chairman
Committee on Appropriations
United States Senate

The Honorable Ron Wyden
Chair
The Honorable Mike Crapo
Ranking Member Committee on Finance
United States Senate

The Honorable Patty Murray
Chair
The Honorable Richard Burr
Ranking Member
Committee on Health, Education, Labor, and Pensions
United States Senate

The Honorable Gary C. Peters
Chairman
The Honorable Rob Portman
Ranking Member
Committee on Homeland Security and Governmental Affairs
United States Senate

The Honorable Kyrsten Sinema
Chair
The Honorable James Lankford
Ranking Member
Subcommittee on Government Operations and Border Management
Committee on Homeland Security and Governmental Affairs
United States Senate

The Honorable Rosa L. DeLauro
Chair
The Honorable Kay Granger
Ranking Member
Committee on Appropriations
House of Representatives

The Honorable Frank Pallone, Jr.
Chair
The Honorable Cathy McMorris Rodgers
Republican Leader
Committee on Energy and Commerce
House of Representatives

The Honorable Bennie G. Thompson
Chair
The Honorable John Katko
Ranking Member
Committee on Homeland Security
House of Representatives

The Honorable Carolyn B. Maloney
Chairwoman
The Honorable James Comer
Ranking Member
Committee on Oversight and Reform
House of Representatives

The Honorable Peter A. DeFazio
Chair
The Honorable Sam Graves
Ranking Member
Committee on Transportation and Infrastructure
House of Representatives

The Honorable Garret Graves
Ranking Member
Subcommittee on Aviation
Committee on Transportation and Infrastructure
House of Representatives

The Honorable Richard Neal
Chair
The Honorable Kevin Brady
Republican Leader
Committee on Ways and Means
House of Representatives

Appendix I: Objectives, Scope, and Methodology

This report addresses (1) the effects of the COVID-19 pandemic on selected aviation and aerospace industry sectors; (2) the actions, if any, that selected stakeholders took in response; (3) actions the Federal Aviation Administration took to help the aviation industry respond to the pandemic, and selected aviation stakeholders' perspectives on those actions; and (4) the outlook for aviation industry recovery, and stakeholder considerations for potential federal support in assisting the aviation industry in the future.

To identify the effects of the pandemic on selected aviation industry sectors, we analyzed Department of Transportation (DOT) Form 41 financial and operational data for calendar years 2019 and 2020—the most recent and complete data available. All dollar figures in this report are nominal unless otherwise noted. To assess the reliability of these data, we reviewed the quality control procedures used by DOT and subsequently determined that the data were sufficiently reliable for our purposes. We also analyzed financial statements reported to the Securities and Exchange Commission by publicly-traded airlines and other aviation businesses from the first quarter through the fourth quarter of 2020 to obtain quantitative information on their financial performance as well as qualitative descriptions of the impact of the pandemic on businesses and actions those businesses took in response.[1] We reported on

[1] The four quarters cover the 12 months of calendar year 2020.

the immediate effects of the pandemic based on the expectation that other effects will be long-term.

We conducted interviews about the effects of the COVID-19 pandemic on selected aviation and aerospace industry sectors and actions stakeholders took in response with a judgmental sample of 47 aviation and aerospace industry stakeholders, including six passenger airlines (two network, two low-cost, and two regional airlines); three cargo airlines; 11 large and medium hub airports; five airframe, engine, or aerostructures manufacturers; three repair stations that provide aircraft maintenance, repair, and overhaul services; two commercial space launch providers; two aviation labor organizations; one engineering and analytics firm; three credit rating agencies; two aviation industry analysts; and nine industry associations. We selected stakeholders to represent a cross-section of sectors within the aviation and aerospace industries as well as based on geographic representation. Because we used a judgmental sample of industry stakeholders, findings from these interviews cannot be generalized to a broader population. However, we determined that the selection of these stakeholders was appropriate for our design and objectives and that these interviews would generate valid and reliable evidence to support our work. See Table 2 for the list of stakeholders we interviewed.

Table 2. Selected aviation and aerospace industry stakeholders GAO interviewed

U.S. federal agencies
Department of Transportation
Federal Aviation Administration
Analytics and engineering firms
BryceTech, LLC
Industry associations
Aeronautical Repair Station Association
Aerospace Industries Association
Aircraft Owners and Pilots Association
Airports Council International–North America
American Association of Airport Executives
Commercial Spaceflight Federation
General Aviation Manufacturers Association
National Business Aviation Association
Satellite Industry Association
Aviation labor organizations
Airline Pilots Association
International Association of Machinists and Aerospace Workers

Table 2. Continued.

Passenger airlines
American Airlines
Delta Air Lines
Frontier Airlines
Spirit Airlines
SkyWest Airlines
Mesa Airlines
Cargo airlines
United Parcel Service
Western Global Airlines
USA Jet Airlines
Aviation manufacturers
Boeing
GE Aviation
Gulfstream Aerospace
Spirit AeroSystems
Textron Aviation
Repair station operators
Aviation Technical Services
HAECO Americas
Velocity Aerospace
Large and medium hub airports
Baltimore/Washington Thurgood Marshall International Airport
Bradley International Airport
Chicago O'Hare International Airport
Cleveland-Hopkins International Airport
Dallas-Fort Worth International Airport
Denver International Airport
Hartsfield-Jackson Atlanta International Airport
Nashville International Airport
Norman Y. Mineta San Jose International Airport
Pittsburgh International Airport
St. Louis Lambert International Airport
Commercial space launch providers
Blue Origin
Space-X
Credit rating agencies
Fitch Ratings
Moody's Investors Service
S&P Global Ratings
Aviation industry analysts
Helane Becker, Cowen Group
William Swelbar, Swelbar–Zhong Consultancy

Source: GAO. | GAO 22-104429.

Survey of Smaller Airports

To identify the effects of the COVID-19 pandemic on smaller airports (i.e., small hub, non-hub, non-primary commercial service, general aviation, and reliever airports), and actions those airports took in response, we designed and administered a web-based survey of a stratified random sample of smaller airports from November 16, 2020, to December 11, 2020.

Survey Population and Sample Design

We constructed the population of airports for our survey sample using data on existing and proposed airports from the Federal Aviation Administration's 2019-2023 National Plan of Integrated Airport Systems (NPIAS), the most recent version available when we began our audit work. Using NPIAS data, we determined that there were (1) 380 primary airports—including 30 large hub, 31 medium hub, 72 small hub, and 247 non-hub airports; (2) 2,941 non-primary airports—including 126 non- primary commercial service airports, 2,554 general aviation airports, and 261 reliever airports;[2] and (3) 7 proposed airports. We excluded from this population large hub and medium airports, non-primary airports with an unclassified role, airports outside of the continental U.S., and proposed airports. The outcome was a survey sample frame of 2,752 airports that included 64 small hub airports, 209 non-hub airports, 63 non-primary commercial service airports, and 2,416 general aviation and reliever airports.

Table 3. Description of the sample frame, stratification, and sample sizes for the stratified random sample of smaller airports

Stratum	Population size	Sample size	Number of completed surveys
Small hub	64	64	59
Non-hub	209	209	183
Non-primary commercial service	63	63	61
General aviation and reliever	2,416	800	514
Total	2,752	1,136	817

Source: GAO, based on analysis of Federal Aviation Administration data. | GAO-22-104429.
Note: Small hub, non-hub, and non-primary commercial service airports were selected with certainty.

We selected a stratified random sample of 1,136 airports that included 64 small hub airports, 209 non-hub airports, 63 non-primary commercial airports,

[2] Non-primary airports are categorized as either national, regional, local, basic, or unclassified.

and 800 general aviation and reliever airports. Small hub, non- hub, and non-primary commercial service airports were selected with certainty. To determine the appropriate sample size for the general aviation and reliever airports, we determined the minimum sample size needed to achieve precision levels of percentage estimates within plus or minus 5 percentage points. We then increased this sample size for an expected response rate of 64 percent in order to achieve the necessary number of completed surveys for our desired precision level (see Table 3). We obtained completed questionnaires from 817 respondents, or about a 72 percent unweighted response rate. The weighted response rate was 65 percent. The survey results can be generalized to the target population of 2,752 smaller airports.

Administration of Survey and Quality Assurance

We developed a questionnaire to obtain information about the effects of the COVID-19 pandemic on smaller airports, and the actions these airports took in response. On November 9, 2020, we sent an initial email alerting airport contacts to the upcoming web-based survey, and a week later, the web-based survey was also delivered to recipients via email message. Our email message described the purpose and topic of the survey, and encouraged the respondent to consult with other individuals in the provider's organization if that would increase the accuracy of their responses. The web-based survey requested information on, among other things, the effects of the pandemic on scheduled commercial passenger air service and airport revenue streams; changes in airport operating expenses and capital improvement projects; the outlook for businesses operating on airport property including repair stations, fixed base operators, pilot schools, aviation maintenance technician schools, and concessions; and airport use of CARES Act grant funding. To help increase our response rate, we sent reminder emails on December 3 and December 8, 2020 and called airport contacts. The survey was available from November 16 through December 11, 2020. Our survey included both closed-ended and open-ended questions. We performed a content analysis on select open-ended questions, whereby one analyst coded all comments using a list of developed categories, and a second analyst independently coded the first 100 responses for each selected question, then reviewed the remaining assigned codes for selected questions as a quality assurance step.

To pretest the questionnaire, we conducted interviews with officials from eight airports with knowledge about their airport's operations. Each pretest was conducted on the phone. We selected pretest respondents to represent a range of airport categories in different parts of the country. We conducted these pretests to determine if the questions were burdensome, understandable, and measured what we intended, and to ensure we could identify an appropriate individual who was knowledgeable about their airport operations to respond to the survey. On the basis of feedback from the pretests, we modified the questions as appropriate.

Sampling Error and Estimation

To produce the estimates from this survey, answers from each responding case were weighted in the analysis to generalize to the members of the population, including those who were not selected or did not respond to the survey. Estimates produced from this sample are generalizable to the target population of 2,752 smaller airports.

Because our results are based on a sample and different samples could provide different estimates, we express our confidence in the precision of our particular sample's results as a 95 percent confidence interval. We are 95 percent confident that each of the confidence intervals in this report include the true values in the study population. Unless we note otherwise, percentage estimates based on all airports have 95 percent confidence intervals of within plus or minus 10 percentage points.

Non-Sampling Error

In addition to the reported sampling errors, the practical difficulties of conducting any survey may introduce other types of errors, commonly referred to as non-sampling errors. For example, differences in how a particular question is interpreted, the sources of information available to respondents, or the types of people who do not respond can introduce unwanted variability into the survey results. We included steps in both the data collection and data analysis stages for the purpose of minimizing such non-sampling errors.

We took the following steps to increase the response rate: pre-testing the questionnaires with airports, and conducting multiple follow-ups to identify the appropriate contact at some airports and to encourage responses to the survey.

Survey Analysis

We analyzed the response status to our survey to identify potential sources of nonresponse bias, in accordance with best practices in survey research and echoed in Office of Management and Budget, Standards and Guidelines for Statistical Surveys (September 2006). We examined the response propensity of the sampled airports using both bivariate and multivariate logistic regression models. The factors we examined included airport characteristics available for respondents and non-respondents on the NPIAS sample frame: airport ownership, role, the number of revenue passengers that boarded aircraft (enplanements), the 5-year estimate of airport improvements eligible for federal development grants under the Airport Improvement Program, the number of aircraft hangered or based at the airport, and the stratification variable that combined hub and airport category. We detected significant associations between the probability of response and the stratification variable, role, enplanements, and number of based aircraft.

We adjusted for the characteristics significantly associated with response propensity using weighting class adjustments. Specifically, we grouped the predicted response propensity derived from our logistic regression model using quintiles of the predicted response propensity distribution to form five weighting adjustment groups. We applied nonresponse adjustments to the sampling weights within these groups to form nonresponse-adjusted analysis weights used in our survey analyses.

The nonresponse bias analysis and subsequent weighted adjustments only included variables available on the NPIAS sample frame and did not account for unobserved variables that could potentially be related to the likelihood of response. However, based on our knowledge of aviation operations, we did not expect survey responses or the likelihood of response to vary by other airport characteristics. Based on this nonresponse bias analysis and resulting nonresponse-adjusted analysis weights, we determined that estimates using these weights are generalizable to the population of smaller airports and are sufficiently reliable for the purposes of our reporting objectives.

We compared—as appropriate—weighted survey estimates generated by the airport strata described above. For each subgroup, we produced percentage estimates and standard errors for each level and used these results to confirm the significance of the differences between weighted survey estimates.

To identify the actions the Federal Aviation Administration (FAA) took to help the aviation industry respond to the pandemic, we reviewed requests for regulatory relief submitted to FAA by aviation stakeholders and FAA's regulatory rulemakings, exemptions, and extensions, as well as operational guidance. We interviewed officials from FAA divisions responsible for implementing these actions as well as those of the 47 aviation and aerospace stakeholders selected whose operations were potentially affected by these actions.

To describe the outlook for aviation industry recovery and stakeholder considerations for potential federal support in assisting the aviation industry in the future, we reviewed forecasts published by aviation industry stakeholders, including consulting firms, credit rating agencies, and an aviation manufacturer, and synthesized their findings. We also interviewed the 47 aviation and aerospace industry stakeholders to obtain their perspectives on considerations for federal assistance, and reviewed our prior work on civil aviation and federal assistance to the private sector.

We conducted this performance audit from July 2020 through October 2021 in accordance with generally accepted government auditing standards. Those standards require that we plan and perform the audit to obtain sufficient, appropriate evidence to provide a reasonable basis for our findings and conclusions based on our audit objectives. We believe that the evidence obtained provides a reasonable basis for our findings and conclusions based on our audit objectives.

Appendix II: Survey of Smaller Airports

This appendix contains selected questions from our survey of smaller airports and their responses. Our web-based survey of a stratified random sample of small hub, non-hub, non-primary commercial service, and general aviation and reliever airports was administered from November 16, 2020 to December 11, 2020. Our survey was comprised of two types of questions: those for which several possible answers were provided to choose from (closed-ended) and those that allowed respondents to provide their own answers (open-ended). We did not verify the statements of those who completed the survey. In this appendix, we include selected survey questions and aggregate results of responses to both closed-ended and open-ended questions. Using professional judgment, we excluded some survey questions from our analysis due to the timing of our survey field period and report issuance. The survey results for the closed-ended questions were weighted in our analysis to be generalizable to the members of our target population of 2,752 smaller airports, including those who were not selected or that did not respond to our survey. General aviation and reliever airports made up the majority (about 88 percent) of smaller airports (see Table 4). For all questions that ask for a comparison between 2019 and 2020, the respondent was presented with a range of options, including: (1) decrease by 76-100%, 51-75%, 26-50%, 10-25%, or less than 10%; (2) about the same (roughly 0%); and (3) increase by more than 100%, 76-100%, 51-75%, 26-50%, 10-25%, or less than 10%. In our analysis, we collapsed the response categories in order to produce statistically reliable estimates. For selected open-ended questions, we performed a non-generalizable content analysis of written responses. For a detailed discussion of our survey methodologies, see appendix I.

Results for the generalizable, closed-ended questions are presented below with lower and upper bounds for 95 percent confidence intervals. We have noted where the margin of error between the estimate and the upper or lower bound is greater than 10 or 20 percentage points:

- Superscript "a": The margin of error between the estimate and the upper or lower bound is greater than 10 percentage points, and therefore should be interpreted with caution.
- DNR (data not reliable): The margin of error between the estimate and upper or lower bound is greater than 20 percentage points and was considered unreliable; these estimates were not included in our findings.

Table 4. The population size and distribution of smaller airports by survey strata

Strata	Population size	Percent
Small hub	64	2
Non-hub	209	8
Non-primary commercial service	63	2
General aviation/reliever	2,416	88
Total	2,752	100

Source: GAO, based on analysis of Federal Aviation Administration data. | GAO-22-104429.

Survey of Smaller Airports

Is scheduled commercial passenger air service provided at your airport?

Estimated percentage (lower bound, upper bound)					
Response	Total	Small hub	Non-hub	Non-primary commercial service	General aviation/ reliever
Yes	14 (13, 15)	100 (95, 100)	97 (93, 99)	93 (84, 98)	2 (1,4)
No	86 (85, 87)	0 (0, 5)	3 (1, 7)	7 (2, 16)	98 (96,99)

A. If yes, what was the estimated change in scheduled commercial passenger air service, as measured by enplanements, when comparing the following months from 2019 and 2020?

April 2019 vs April 2020

Estimated percentage (lower bound, upper bound)					
Response	Total	Small hub	Non-hub	Non-primary commercial service	General aviation/ reliever
Decrease					
>50%	90 (85, 93)	97 (88, 100)	94 (89,97)	85 (73, 94)[a]	DNR
1-50%	8 (4, 12)	3 (0, 12)	5 (2, 10)	7 (2, 18)[a]	DNR
Roughly 0%	2 (0, 5)	0 (0, 5)	0 (0, 2)	4 (0, 13)	DNR
Increase	0 (0,2)	0 (0, 5)	1 (0, 3)	0 (0, 5)	DNR
Don't know	1 (0, 2)	0 (0, 5)	0 (0, 2)	4 (0, 13)	DNR

September 2019 versus September 2020

Estimated percentage (lower bound, upper bound)					
Response	Total	Small hub	Non-hub	Non-primary commercial service	General aviation/reliever
Decrease					
>50%	64 (60, 69)	77 (65, 87)	69 (66,71)	53 (50, 55)	DNR
1-50%	31 (27, 35)	23 (13, 35)	28 (26, 31)	38 (25, 52)[a]	DNR
Roughly 0%	2 (1, 6)	0 (0, 5)	1 (0, 4)	2 (0, 10)	DNR
Increase	1 (0, 4)	0 (0, 5)	2 (0, 5)	4 (0, 13)	DNR
Don't know	1 (0, 2)	0 (0, 5)	0 (0, 2)	4 (0, 13)	DNR

Is unscheduled/charter air service provided at your airport?

Estimated percentage (lower bound, upper bound)					
Response	Total	Small hub	Non-hub	Non-primary commercial service	General aviation/reliever
Yes	35 (32, 39)	78 (65, 88)	75 (72, 77)	62 (60, 64)	30 (27, 34)
No	65 (61, 68)	22 (12, 35)	25 (23, 28)	38 (36, 40)	70 (66, 73)

A. If yes, what was the estimated change in unscheduled/charter air service, as measured by enplanements, when comparing the following months from 2019 and 2020?

April 2019 vs April 2020

Estimated percentage (lower bound, upper bound)					
Response	Total	Small hub	Non-hub	Non-primary commercial service	General aviation/reliever
Decrease	67 (62, 72)	72 (57, 84)[a]	79 (71, 85)	58 (41, 74)[a]	64 (58, 71)
Roughly 0%	15 (11, 20)	11 (4, 24)[a]	10 (5, 16)	16 (6, 31)[a]	17 (11, 23)
Increase	7 (5, 11)	4 (1, 15)[a]	2 (1, 6)	5 (1, 18)[a]	9 (5, 14)
Don't know	11 (8, 15)	13 (5, 26)[a]	9 (5, 15)	21 (10, 37)[a]	11 (6, 16)

September 2019 vs. September 2020

Estimated percentage (lower bound, upper bound)					
Response	Total	Small hub	Non-hub	Non-primary commercial service	General aviation/reliever
Decrease	58 (53, 63)	70 (54, 82)[a]	72 (69, 74)	50 (47, 53)	55 (47, 62)
Roughly 0%	19 (14, 23)	11 (4, 24)[a]	10 (6, 17)	18 (8, 34)[a]	21 (15, 28)
Increase	12 (9, 16)	7 (1, 18)[a]	9 (5, 15)	11 (3, 25)[a]	14 (9, 20)
Don't know	11 (8, 15)	13 (5, 26)[a]	9 (5, 15)	21 (10, 37)[a]	11 (6, 17)

Is non-mail cargo air service provided at your airport?

Estimated percentage (lower bound, upper bound)					
Response	Total	Small hub	Non-hub	Non-primary commercial service	General aviation/reliever
Yes	13 (11, 15)	81 (69, 90)[a]	49 (47, 52)	40 (38, 42)	7 (5, 10)
No	87 (85, 89)	19 (10, 31)[a]	51 (48, 53)	60 (58, 62)	93 (90, 95)

A. If yes, what was the estimated change in non-mail cargo air service, as measured by weight (either pounds or tonnage), when comparing the following months from 2019 and 2020?

April 2019 vs April 2020

Estimated percentage (lower bound, upper bound)					
Response	Total	Small hub	Non-hub	Non-primary commercial service	General aviation/reliever
Decrease	36 (30, 43)	54 (50, 58)	42 (39, 46)	DNR	29 (16, 46)[a]
Roughly 0%	35 (28, 42)	15 (6, 28)[a]	27 (18, 37)[a]	DNR	42 (26, 59)[a]
Increase	15 (10, 21)	31 (19, 46)[a]	15 (8, 24)	13 (3, 32)[a]	11 (3, 25)[a]
Don't know	14 (9, 20)	0 (0, 6)	16 (9, 25)	8 (1, 27)[a]	18 (7, 33)[a]

September 2019 vs September 2020

Estimated percentage (lower bound, upper bound)					
Response	Total	Small hub	Non-hub	Non-primary commercial service	General aviation/reliever
Decrease	26 (19, 32)	30 (17, 45)[a]	22 (14, 32)[a]	DNR	28 (14, 45)[a]
Roughly 0%	33 (26, 40)	15 (6, 28)[a]	29 (26, 33)	DNR	37 (22, 54)[a]
Increase	27 (22, 33)	55 (51, 59)	33 (29, 36)	DNR	17 (7, 32)[a]
Don't know	14 (9, 21)	0 (0, 6)	16 (9, 25)	8 (1, 27)[a]	18 (8, 34)[a]

Are there general aviation operations at your airport?

(General aviation operations may include business jet operations, turboprops, piston airplanes, or helicopters. Please do not include military operations in your response.)

Estimated percentage (lower bound, upper bound)					
Response	Total	Small hub	Non-hub	Non-primary commercial service	General aviation/reliever
Yes	95 (93, 96)	98 (91, 100)	99 (97, 100)	100 (95, 100)	94 (92, 96)
No	5 (4, 7)	2 (0, 9)	1 (0, 3)	0 (0, 5)	6 (4, 8)

A. If yes, what was the estimated change in general aviation operations when comparing the following months from 2019 and 2020?

April 2019 vs April 2020

Estimated percentage (lower bound, upper bound)					
Response	Total	Small hub	Non-hub	Non-primary commercial service	General aviation/reliever
Decrease					
>50%	29 (26, 32)	52 (48, 55)	41 (39, 44)	36 (24, 49)[a]	27 (24, 31)
1-50%	40 (36, 43)	38 (34, 41)	40 (38, 43)	38 (36, 40)	40 (36, 44)
Roughly 0%	18 (15, 21)	2 (0, 9)	7 (4, 11)	11 (5, 22)[a]	20 (16, 23)
Increase	8 (6, 10)	7 (2, 17)	6 (3, 11)	7 (2, 16)	8 (6, 11)
Don't know	5 (4, 7)	2 (0, 9)	6 (3, 10)	8 (3, 18)	5 (3, 7)

September 2019 vs September 2020

Estimated percentage (lower bound, upper bound)					
Response	Total	Small hub	Non-hub	Non-primary commercial service	General aviation/reliever
Decrease					
>50%	14 (12, 17)	5 (1, 14)	17 (12, 23)	20 (11, 32)[a]	14 (11, 17)
1-50%	42 (39, 46)	60 (57, 64)	44 (42, 47)	41 (39, 43)	41 (38, 45)
Roughly 0%	21 (18, 24)	9 (3, 19)[a]	8 (4, 13)	11 (5, 22)[a]	23 (19, 26)
Increase	17 (15, 20)	24 (14, 37)[a]	25 (23, 27)	20 (11, 32)[a]	17 (14, 19)
Don't know	5 (4, 7)	2 (0, 9)	6 (3, 10)	8 (3, 18)	5 (3, 8)

What was the estimated change in your airport's aeronautical operating revenue, when comparing the months of September 2019 versus September 2020?

Estimated percentage (lower bound, upper bound)					
Response	Total	Small hub	Non-hub	Non-primary commercial service	General aviation/ reliever
Decrease					
>50%	14 (12, 17)	30 (19, 44)[a]	38 (36, 41)	15 (7, 26)[a]	12 (9, 15)
1-50%	44 (40, 47)	54 (51, 58)	54 (51, 57)	54 (52, 56)	42 (38, 46)
Roughly 0%	28 (25, 31)	5 (1, 14)	2 (0, 5)	18 (9, 30)[a]	31 (27, 34)
Increase	9 (7, 11)	10 (4, 21)[a]	6 (3, 10)	10 (4, 20)[a]	10 (7, 13)
Don't know	5 (4, 7)	0 (0, 5)	1 (0, 3)	3 (0, 11)	6 (4, 8)

What was the estimated change in your airport's Passenger Facility Charges (PFCs), when comparing the months of September 2019 versus September 2020?

(If your airport does not collect PFCs, please select "not applicable.")

Estimated percentage (lower bound, upper bound)					
Response	Total	Small hub	Non-hub	Non-primary commercial service	General aviation/reliever
Decrease	64 (57, 70)	93 (83, 98)	97 (93, 99)	79 (62, 91)[a]	25 (14, 40)[a]
Roughly 0%	28 (22, 35)	2 (0, 9)	1 (0, 4)	12 (3, 27)[a]	60 (45, 74)[a]
Increase	3 (1, 6)	3 (0, 12)	0 (0, 2)	6 (1, 20)[a]	5 (1, 15)[a]
Don't know	5 (3, 10)	2 (0, 9)	2 (0, 5)	3 (0, 15)[a]	10 (3, 22)[a]

What was the estimated change in your airport's non-aeronautical operating revenue, when comparing the months of September 2019 versus September 2020?

Estimated percentage (lower bound, upper bound)					
Response	Total	Small hub	Non-hub	Non-primary commercial service	General aviation/reliever
Decrease					
>50%	10 (8, 12)	47 (44, 51)	32 (30, 34)	13 (6, 24)[a]	7 (5, 9)
1-50%	20 (17, 22)	48 (44, 51)	54 (51, 57)	31 (20, 44)[a]	16 (13, 19)
Roughly 0%	51 (48, 55)	3 (0, 12)	8 (4, 13)	39 (37, 42)	57 (53, 61)
Increase	4 (3, 5)	0 (0, 5)	5 (2, 9)	7 (2, 16)	4 (2, 6)
Don't know	15 (13, 18)	2 (0, 9)	1 (0, 4)	10 (4, 20)[a]	17 (14, 20)

Does your airport have non-aeronautical land leases?

Estimated percentage (lower bound, upper bound)					
Response	Total	Small hub	Non-hub	Non-primary commercial service	General aviation/reliever
Yes	47 (43, 50)	91 (81, 97)[a]	76 (74, 78)	70 (57, 81)[a]	42 (38, 46)
No	53 (50, 57)	9 (3, 19)[a]	24 (22, 26)	30 (19, 43)[a]	58 (54, 62)

Have any measures been taken to generate additional revenue at your airport since the start of the COVID-19 pandemic?

Estimated percentage (lower bound, upper bound)					
Response	Total	Small hub	Non-hub	Non-primary commercial service	General aviation/reliever
Yes	26 (24, 29)	61 (58, 65)	45 (42, 48)	26 (16, 39)[a]	24 (21, 27)
No	74 (71, 76)	39 (35, 42)	55 (52, 58)	74 (61, 84)[a]	76 (73, 79)

A. If yes, please describe any measures taken to generate additional revenue.

Identified revenue measures	Number of responses
Built or developed revenue opportunities (built structures to rent out, developed land for lease, etc.)	59
Filled office or land vacancies (empty, available resources were filled with rent-paying tenants)	62
Increased marketing (additional advertising/marketing efforts to raise awareness about opportunities to bring business to the airport)	37

Identified revenue measures	Number of responses
Opportunistic and/or temporary measures (revenue-generating activities taking advantage of low activity at airport, adapting to COVID-19 precautions, etc., that are likely to be discontinued once aviation recovers)	26
Created incentives (efforts that would directly encourage or drive demand, through promos, discounts, etc.)	29
Raised rates and/or fees	18
Pursued favorable agreements (airports worked to gain greater efficiency with their agreements/pursuing more favorable terms for themselves, e.g., tenants with lower rates, renegotiated contracts)	17
Sold assets (airports sold off land or other assets in order to raise revenue)	7

Note: The above results are based on a content analysis of written responses. A total of 249 respondents provided a valid, written response to this question. Respondents may have mentioned more than one measure taken, therefore responses do not add up to 100 percent. There were also 60 comments made regarding airport revenue measures that did not fall into the identified categories.

Have any of the following measures been taken to reduce operating costs at your airport since the start of the COVID-19 pandemic?

A. Hiring freezes

Estimated percentage (lower bound, upper bound)					
Response	Total	Small hub	Non-hub	Non-primary commercial service	General aviation/ reliever
Yes	29 (26, 32)	75 (62, 85)[a]	57 (54, 59)	38 (36, 41)	25 (22, 28)
No	46 (43, 49)	24 (14, 37)[a]	41 (39, 44)	55 (53, 57)	47 (43, 51)
Don't know	0 (0, 1)	0 (0, 5)	0 (0, 2)	0 (0, 5)	0 (0, 1)
Not applicable	25 (22, 28)	2 (0, 9)	2 (0, 5)	7 (2, 16)	28 (24, 31)

B. Staff layoffs

Estimated percentage (lower bound, upper bound)					
Response	Total	Small hub	Non-hub	Non-primary commercial service	General aviation/ reliever
Yes	6 (5, 8)	19 (10, 31)[a]	14 (10, 20)	3 (0, 12)	5 (3, 7)
No	72 (69, 75)	80 (67, 89)[a]	84 (78, 89)	92 (82, 97)[a]	70 (67, 74)
Don't know	0 (0, 1)	0 (0, 5)	0 (0, 2)	0 (0, 5)	0 (0, 2)
Not applicable	21 (18, 24)	2 (0, 9)	2 (0, 5)	5 (1, 14)	24 (21, 27)

C. Reduce staff hours

Estimated percentage (lower bound, upper bound)					
Response	Total	Small hub	Non-hub	Non-primary commercial service	General aviation/ reliever
Yes	20 (17, 22)	39 (35, 42)	34 (32, 37)	22 (12, 34)[a]	18 (15, 21)
No	61 (58, 64)	56 (52, 60)	66 (63, 68)	73 (60, 84)[a]	60 (57, 64)
Don't know	0 (0, 1)	0 (0, 5)	0 (0, 2)	0 (0, 5)	0 (0, 1)
Not applicable	19 (16, 22)	5 (1, 14)	0 (0, 2)	5 (1, 14)	21 (18, 25)

D. Reduce staff travel

Estimated percentage (lower bound, upper bound)					
Response	Total	Small hub	Non-hub	Non-primary commercial service	General aviation/ reliever
Yes	44 (41, 48)	98 (91, 100)	88 (83, 93)	75 (62, 85)[a]	38 (34, 42)
No	29 (26, 32)	0 (0, 5)	10 (6, 16)	20 (11, 32)[a]	31 (28, 35)
Don't know	0 (0, 1)	0 (0, 5)	0 (0, 2)	2 (0, 9)	0 (0, 1)
Not applicable	27 (23, 30)	2 (0, 9)	1 (0, 4)	3 (0, 12)	30 (27, 34)

E. Reduce staff training

Estimated percentage (lower bound, upper bound)					
Response	Total	Small hub	Non-hub	Non-primary commercial service	General aviation/ reliever
Yes	26 (23, 29)	47 (44, 51)	54 (51, 56)	36 (24, 49)[a]	23 (20, 26)
No	53 (50, 57)	48 (44, 51)	46 (43, 48)	63 (60, 65)	54 (50, 58)
Don't know	0 (0, 1)	2 (0, 9)	0 (0, 2)	0 (0, 5)	0 (0, 1)
Not applicable	20 (17, 23)	3 (0, 12)	1 (0, 3)	2 (0, 9)	23 (20, 27)

F. Defer debt finance

Estimated percentage (lower bound, upper bound)					
Response	Total	Small hub	Non-hub	Non-primary commercial service	General aviation/ reliever
Yes	3 (2, 5)	8(3, 19)[a]	8 (5, 13)	7 (2, 16)	2 (1, 4)
No	65 (61, 68)	80 (67, 89)[a]	75 (73, 78)	78 (65, 88)[a]	63 (59, 67)
Don't know	4 (3, 5)	2 (0, 9)	2 (1, 6)	5 (1, 14)	4 (2, 6)
Not applicable	29 (25, 32)	10 (4, 21)[a]	14 (9, 20)	10 (4, 21)[a]	31 (27, 35)

G. Defer maintenance

Estimated percentage (lower bound, upper bound)					
Response	Total	Small hub	Non-hub	Non-primary commercial service	General aviation/ reliever
Yes	23 (21, 26)	52 (48, 55)	35 (33, 38)	28 (17, 41)[a]	21 (18, 25)
No	62 (58, 65)	48 (45, 52)	65 (62, 67)	70 (57, 81)[a]	62 (58, 65)
Don't know	1 (0, 2)	0 (0, 5)	0 (0, 2)	0 (0, 5)	1 (0, 2)
Not applicable	14 (11, 17)	0 (0, 5)	0 (0, 2)	2 (0, 9)	16 (13, 19)

H. Other

Estimated percentage (lower bound, upper bound)					
Response	Total	Small hub	Non-hub	Non-primary commercial service	General aviation/ reliever
Yes	9 (6, 12)	49 (44, 53)	24 (16, 34)	8 (1, 26)[a]	6 (4, 10)
No	36 (32, 41)	18 (7, 33)[a]	28 (19, 38)[a]	DNR	37 (32, 43)
Don't know	3 (2, 6)	0 (0, 7)	4 (1, 11)	8 (1, 26)[a]	3 (2, 6)
Not applicable	51 (47, 56)	33 (19, 50)[a]	43 (40, 47)	DNR	53 (48, 58)

Have you made any changes to any ongoing or planned (within the next year) infrastructure/capital improvement projects since the start of the COVID-19 pandemic?

Estimated percentage (lower bound, upper bound)					
Response	Total	Small hub	Non-hub	Non-primary commercial service	General aviation/ reliever
Yes	30 (27, 33)	80 (67, 89)[a]	42 (39, 45)	38 (36, 41)	27 (24, 31)
No	68 (65, 71)	20 (11, 33)[a]	57 (55, 60)	58 (56, 61)	70 (67, 74)
Not applicable	2 (1, 4)	0 (0, 5)	1 (0, 3)	3 (0, 12)	3 (1, 4)

A. If yes, how, if at all, has the scope/timeline for the project(s) been impacted by COVID-19? Please check all that apply.

Project Cancelled

Estimated percentage (lower bound, upper bound)					
Response	Total	Small hub	Non-hub	Non-primary commercial service	General aviation/ reliever
Checked	14 (10, 19)	25 (14, 40)[a]	21 (12, 31)[a]	4 (0, 22)[a]	13 (8, 20)
Not checked	86 (81, 90)	75 (60, 86)[a]	79 (69, 88)[a]	96 (78, 100)[a]	87 (80, 92)

Project Delayed

Estimated percentage (lower bound, upper bound)					
Response	Total	Small hub	Non-hub	Non-primary commercial service	General aviation/ reliever
Checked	77 (72, 82)	92 (80, 98)[a]	77 (66, 86)[a]	DNR	77 (69, 84)
Not checked	23 (18, 28)	8 (2, 20)[a]	23 (14, 34)[a]	DNR	23 (16, 31)

Project Accelerated

Estimated percentage (lower bound, upper bound)					
Response	Total	Small hub	Non-hub	Non-primary commercial service	General aviation/ reliever
Checked	11 (8, 16)	11 (4, 23)[a]	18 (10, 29)[a]	DNR	10 (6, 16)
Not checked	89 (84, 92)	89 (77, 96)[a]	82 (71, 90)[a]	DNR	90 (84, 94)

Other

Estimated percentage (lower bound, upper bound)					
Response	Total	Small hub	Non-hub	Non-primary commercial service	General aviation/ reliever
Checked	7 (5, 11)	6 (1, 18)[a]	10 (5, 19)	DNR	7 (3, 12)
Not checked	93 (89, 95)	94 (82, 99)[a]	90 (81, 95)	DNR	93 (88, 97)

Is your airport at risk of defaulting on any outstanding obligations?

Estimated percentage (lower bound, upper bound)					
Response	Total	Small hub	Non-hub	Non-primary commercial service	General aviation/ reliever
Yes	3 (1, 6)	7 (1, 24)[a]	9 (4, 18)	DNR	1 (0, 6)
No	97 (94, 99)	93 (76, 99)[a]	91 (82, 96)	DNR	99 (94, 100)

Is your airport at risk of closing/ceasing all operations?

Estimated percentage (lower bound, upper bound)					
Response	Total	Small hub	Non-hub	Non-primary commercial service	General aviation/ reliever
Yes	2 (1, 5)	0 (0, 11)[a]	5 (2, 13)	DNR	1 (0, 6)
No	98 (95, 99)	100 (89, 100)[a]	95 (87, 98)	DNR	99 (94, 100)

Do any repair stations operate on your airport's property, whether airport-owned/operated or non-airport owned/operated? (According to FAA, the term "Repair Station" refers to a maintenance facility that has a certificate issued by the FAA under Title 14 of the Code of Federal Regulations (14 C.F.R.) Part 145 and is engaged in the maintenance, inspection, and alteration of aircraft and aircraft products. FAA rules are specific on who can perform maintenance and approve an aircraft, airframe, engines, etc., for return to service after maintenance has been performed.)

Estimated percentage (lower bound, upper bound)					
Response	Total	Small hub	Non-hub	Non-primary commercial service	General aviation/ reliever
Yes	47 (44, 50)	73 (60, 83)[a]	63 (60, 65)	62 (60, 64)	45 (41, 48)
No	53 (50, 56)	27 (17, 40)[a]	37 (35, 40)	38 (36, 40)	55 (52, 59)

A. If yes, if known, how would you describe the overall impact COVID-19 has had on this repair station/these repair stations?

(If more than one business of this type is operating at your airport, please report the overall impact on these businesses at your airport.)

Estimated percentage (lower bound, upper bound)					
Response	Total	Small hub	Non-hub	Non-primary commercial service	General aviation/ reliever
Negative	50 (45, 54)	65 (49, 79)[a]	55 (52, 59)	63 (46, 78)[a]	48 (42, 53)
No impact	25 (21, 29)	12 (4, 25)[a]	13 (7, 20)	21 (10, 37)[a]	27 (22, 32)
Positive	8 (6, 11)	2 (0, 12)	7 (3, 13)	3 (0, 14)[a]	9 (6, 13)
Don't know	17 (14, 21)	21 (10, 36)[a]	25 (17, 34)	13 (4, 28)[a]	16 (12, 22)

Do any fixed base operators (FBOs) operate on your airport's property, whether airport-owned/operated or non-airport owned/operated?

(FBO services may include fueling, hangaring, tie down and parking, aircraft rental, aircraft maintenance, and similar services.)

Estimated percentage (lower bound, upper bound)					
Response	Total	Small hub	Non-hub	Non-primary commercial service	General aviation/reliever
Yes	77 (74, 80)	98 (90, 100)	98 (95, 100)	95 (94, 96)	74 (71, 78)
No	23 (20, 26)	2 (0, 10)	2 (0, 5)	5 (1, 14)	26 (22, 29)

A. If yes, if known, how would you describe the overall impact COVID-19 has had on this FBO/these FBOs?

Estimated percentage (lower bound, upper bound)					
Response	Total	Small hub	Non-hub	Non-primary commercial service	General aviation/ reliever
Very/moderately negative	45 (41, 48)	61 (58, 65)	62 (59, 65)	42 (40, 44)	42 (38, 47)
Slightly negative	30 (27, 34)	23 (13, 36)[a]	24 (22, 27)	28 (17, 42)[a]	31 (27, 35)
No impact	12 (10, 15)	2 (0, 9)	3 (1, 7)	9 (3, 19)[a]	14 (11, 18)
Positive	8 (6, 10)	9 (3, 19)[a]	6 (3, 10)	12 (5, 24)[a]	8 (5, 11)
Don't know	5 (4, 7)	5 (1, 15)	5 (2, 9)	9 (3, 19)[a]	5 (3, 8)

Do any pilot schools operating under Part 141 regulations operate on your airport's property, whether airport-owned/operated or non- airport owned/operated?

(FAA-certificated pilot schools are regulated in accordance with Title 14 of the Code of Federal Regulations (14 C.F.R.) Part 141. Unlike pilot training conducted under 14 C.F.R. Part 61, Part 141 pilot schools are required to use a structured training program and syllabus. Part 141 pilot schools may be able to provide a greater variety of training aids and require dedicated training facilities, flight instructor oversight, and FAA-approved course curricula. Colleges and universities, which may offer aviation degrees, often provide pilot training under Part 141.)

Estimated percentage (lower bound, upper bound)					
Response	Total	Small hub	Non-hub	Non-primary commercial service	General aviation/ reliever
Yes	25 (22, 28)	51 (47, 54)	45 (43, 48)	25 (14, 37)[a]	23 (20, 26)
No	75 (72, 78)	49 (46, 53)	55 (52, 57)	75 (63, 86)[a]	77 (74, 80)

A. If yes, if known, how would you describe the overall impact COVID-19 has had on this school/these schools?

(If more than one business of this type is operating at your airport, please report the overall impact on these businesses at your airport.)

Estimated percentage (lower bound, upper bound)					
Response	Total	Small hub	Non-hub	Non-primary commercial service	General aviation/ reliever
Negative	60 (53, 66)	67 (47, 83)[a]	62 (58, 66)	DNR	59 (51, 66)
No impact	15 (11, 21)	7 (1, 22)[a]	11 (5, 20)	DNR	17 (11, 25)
Positive	13 (9, 19)	17 (6, 35)[a]	11 (5, 19)	DNR	14 (8, 21)
Don't know	11 (8, 16)	10 (2, 27)[a]	16 (9, 26)	DNR	11 (6, 18)

Do any aviation maintenance technician schools operate on your airport's property, whether airport-owned/operated or non-airport owned/operated?

(An Aviation Maintenance Technician School (AMTS) is an educational facility certificated by the FAA to train prospective aircraft mechanics for careers in the airline industry, in aviation maintenance facilities, and in commercial and General Aviation (GA). 14 C.F.R. Part 147 specifies requirements for the certification and operation of an AMTS. The regulation includes both the curriculum requirements and the operating rules for all certificated AMTSs.)

Estimated percentage (lower bound, upper bound)					
Response	Total	Small hub	Non-hub	Non-primary commercial service	General aviation/ reliever
Yes	5 (4, 7)	24 (14, 37)[a]	12 (7, 17)	5 (1, 14)	4 (2, 6)
No	95 (93, 96)	76 (63, 86)[a]	88 (83, 93)	95 (86, 99)	96 (94, 98)

A. If yes, if known, how would you describe the overall impact COVID-19 has had on this school/these schools?

(If more than one business of this type is operating at your airport, please report the overall impact on these businesses at your airport.)

Estimated percentage (lower bound, upper bound)					
Response	Total	Small hub	Non-hub	Non-primary commercial service	General aviation/ reliever
Negative	57 (44, 70)[a]	DNR	DNR	DNR	DNR
No impact	8 (2, 18)[a]	0 (0, 19)[a]	DNR	DNR	DNR
Positive	8 (2, 21)[a]	0 (0, 19)[a]	5 (0, 24)[a]	DNR	DNR
Don't know	28 (16, 42)[a]	DNR	DNR	DNR	DNR

Do any paid parking concessions operate on your airport's property, whether airport-owned/operated or non-airport owned/operated?

Estimated percentage (lower bound, upper bound)					
Response	Total	Small hub	Non-hub	Non-primary commercial service	General aviation/ reliever
Yes	8 (6, 10)	88 (77, 95)[a]	60 (57, 62)	7 (2, 16)	2 (1, 3)
No	92 (90, 94)	12 (5, 23)[a]	40 (38, 43)	93 (84, 98)	98 (97, 99)

A. If yes, if known, how would you describe the overall impact COVID-19 has had on this business?

(If more than one business of this type is operating at your airport, please report the overall impact on these businesses at your airport.)

Estimated percentage (lower bound, upper bound)					
Response	Total	Small hub	Non-hub	Non-primary commercial service	General aviation/ reliever
Negative	91 (82, 96)	98 (90, 100)	99 (95, 100)	DNR	DNR
No impact	8 (3, 17)	0 (0, 6)	0 (0, 3)	DNR	DNR
Positive	0 (0, 3)	0 (0, 6)	1 (0, 5)	DNR	DNR
Don't know	0 (0, 3)	2 (0, 10)	0 (0, 3)	DNR	DNR

Do any car rental or ground transportation concessions operate on your airport's property, whether airport-owned/operated or non- airport owned/operated?

Estimated percentage (lower bound, upper bound)					
Response	Total	Small hub	Non-hub	Non-primary commercial service	General aviation/ reliever
Yes	26 (24, 29)	100 (95, 100)	98 (94, 99)	79 (66, 88)[a]	17 (14, 19)
No	74 (71, 76)	0 (0, 5)	2 (1, 6)	21 (12, 34)[a]	83 (81, 86)

A. If yes, if known, how would you describe the overall impact COVID-19 has had on this business?

(If more than one business of this type is operating at your airport, please report the overall impact on these businesses at your airport.)

Estimated percentage (lower bound, upper bound)					
Response	Total	Small hub	Non-hub	Non-primary commercial service	General aviation/ reliever
Very moderately/ negative	65 (60, 71)	90 (79, 96)[a]	82 (76, 87)	65 (49, 78)[a]	53 (43, 62)
Slightly negative	16 (12, 20)	8 (3, 19)[a]	12 (7, 17)	19 (9, 33)[a]	18 (11, 28)
No impact	6 (3, 10)	0 (0, 5)	0 (0, 2)	2 (0, 11)	11 (5, 19)
Positive	4 (2, 7)	0 (0, 5)	3 (1, 6)	12 (5, 25)[a]	4 (1, 11)
Don't know	9 (5, 13)	2 (0, 9)	3 (1, 7)	2 (0, 11)	13 (7, 22)

Do any food and beverage concessions operate on your airport's property, whether airport-owned/operated or non-airport owned/operated?

Estimated percentage (lower bound, upper bound)					
Response	Total	Small hub	Non-hub	Non-primary commercial service	General aviation/ reliever
Yes	21 (18, 23)	98 (91, 100)	80 (74, 86)	41 (39, 43)	13 (10, 15)
No	79 (77, 82)	2 (0, 9)	20 (14, 26)	59 (57, 61)	87 (85, 90)

A. If yes, if known, how would you describe the overall impact COVID-19 has had on this business?

(If more than one business of this type is operating at your airport, please report the overall impact on these businesses at your airport.)

Estimated percentage (lower bound, upper bound)					
Response	Total	Small hub	Non-hub	Non-primary commercial service	General aviation/ reliever
Very moderately/ negative	89 (84, 93)	98 (91, 100)	94 (89, 97)	88 (69, 97)[a]	85 (75, 93)[a]
Slightly negative	7 (4, 11)	0 (0, 5)	6 (3, 11)	12 (3, 31)[a]	8 (3, 18)
No impact	3 (1, 7)	2 (0, 9)	0 (0, 2)	0 (0, 11)[a]	5 (1, 13)
Positive	1 (0, 4)	0 (0, 5)	0 (0, 2)	0 (0, 11)[a]	1 (0, 8)
Don't know	0 (0, 1)	0 (0, 5)	0 (0, 2)	0 (0, 11)[a]	0 (0, 4)

Do any gift and/or retail concessions operate on your airport's property, whether airport-owned/operated or non-airport owned/operated?

Estimated percentage (lower bound, upper bound)					
Response	Total	Small hub	Non-hub	Non-primary commercial service	General aviation/reliever
Yes	9 (7, 11)	100 (95, 100)	39 (36, 41)	3 (0, 11)	4 (2, 6)
No	91 (89, 93)	0 (0, 5)	61 (59, 64)	97 (89, 100)	96 (94, 98)

A. If yes, if known, how would you describe the overall impact COVID-19 has had on this business?

(If more than one business of this type is operating at your airport, please report the overall impact on these businesses at your airport.)

Estimated percentage (lower bound, upper bound)					
Response	Total	Small hub	Non-hub	Non-primary commercial service	General aviation/ reliever
Negative	92 (82, 97)	100 (95, 100)	100 (96, 100)	DNR	DNR
No impact	4 (1, 12)	0 (0, 5)	0 (0, 4)	DNR	DNR
Positive	2 (0, 9)	0 (0, 5)	0 (0, 4)	DNR	DNR
Don't know	2 (0, 11)	0 (0, 5)	0 (0, 4)	DNR	DNR

Do any other aviation-related businesses operate on your airport's property, whether airport-owned/operated or non-airport owned/operated?

Estimated percentage (lower bound, upper bound)					
Response	Total	Small hub	Non-hub	Non-primary commercial service	General aviation/ reliever
Yes	34 (31, 37)	56 (52, 59)	35 (33, 38)	38 (36, 41)	33 (30, 37)
No	66 (63, 69)	44 (41, 48)	65 (62, 67)	62 (59, 64)	67 (63, 70)

A. If yes, if known, how would you describe the overall impact COVID-19 has had on this business?

(If more than one business of this type is operating at your airport, please report the overall impact on these businesses at your airport.)

Estimated percentage (lower bound, upper bound)					
Response	Total	Small hub	Non-hub	Non-primary commercial service	General aviation/ reliever
Negative	54 (48, 60)	70 (51, 84)[a]	61 (56, 65)	DNR	53 (47, 60)
No impact	26 (21, 31)	6 (1, 20)[a]	17 (9, 29)[a]	DNR	27 (21, 33)
Positive	7 (4, 11)	12 (3, 28)[a]	11 (5, 22)[a]	DNR	6 (3, 11)
Don't know	13 (9, 18)	12 (3, 28)[a]	11 (5, 21)[a]	9 (1, 28)[a]	13 (9, 19)

Have you provided any rent or other rent relief to any of the tenants operating at your airport?

Estimated percentage (lower bound, upper bound)					
Response	Total	Small hub	Non-hub	Non-primary commercial service	General aviation/ reliever
Yes	23 (21, 26)	81 (69, 90)[a]	78 (76, 80)	44 (42, 47)	16 (13, 19)
No	77 (74, 79)	19 (10, 31)[a]	22 (20, 24)	56 (53, 58)	84 (81, 87)

A. If yes, please describe the type of relief you have provided to tenants.

Identified relief measures	Number of responses
Deferred payments (airports provided relief to tenants by not holding tenants to payment deadlines for a period of time, allowing them to catch up on what they owed later on (by a specified future date)	152
Waived payments (airports provided relief to tenants by providing abatement/cancellation/waiver of rent, MAG, or fees for an amount of time)	117
Changed rates and/or agreements (reduced rates and fees, changed/adjusted leases and agreements, opted not to proceed with rate increases, etc.)	77
Other relief measures	26

Note: The above results are based on a content analysis of written responses. A total of 289 respondents provided a valid, written response to this question. Respondents may have mentioned more than one measure taken, therefore responses do not add up to 100 percent.

Have any of your tenant businesses defaulted on any rents?

Estimated percentage (lower bound, upper bound)					
Response	Total	Small hub	Non-hub	Non-primary commercial service	General aviation/ reliever
Yes	10 (8, 12)	27 (17, 40)[a]	30 (28, 33)	20 (11, 32)[a]	7 (5, 10)
No	90 (88, 92)	73 (60, 83)[a]	70 (67, 72)	80 (68, 89)[a]	93 (90, 95)

Has your airport received a CARES Act Airport Grant?

Estimated percentage (lower bound, upper bound)					
Response	Total	Small hub	Non-hub	Non-primary commercial service	General aviation/ reliever
Yes	91 (88, 93)	100 (95, 100)	100 (98, 100)	100 (95, 100)	89 (86, 92)
No	9 (7, 12)	0 (0, 5)	0 (0, 2)	0 (0, 5)	11 (8, 14)

A. If yes, as of October 2020, for what purposes have you used or do you intend to use the grant award?

Payroll/labor costs

Estimated percentage (lower bound, upper bound)					
Response	Total	Small hub	Non-hub	Non-primary commercial service	General aviation/ reliever
Checked	47 (43, 50)	85 (73, 93)[a]	82 (76, 87)	69 (56, 80)[a]	42 (37, 46)
Not checked	53 (50, 57)	15 (7, 27)[a]	18 (13, 24)	31 (20, 44)[a]	58 (54, 63)

Utilities

Estimated percentage (lower bound, upper bound)					
Response	Total	Small hub	Non-hub	Non-primary commercial service	General aviation/reliever
Checked	35 (31, 38)	46 (42, 49)	60 (57, 62)	46 (44, 48)	32 (28, 35)
Not checked	65 (62, 69)	54 (51, 58)	40 (38, 43)	54 (52, 56)	68 (65, 72)

Debt Service

Estimated percentage (lower bound, upper bound)					
Response	Total	Small hub	Non-hub	Non-primary commercial service	General aviation/ reliever
Checked	12 (10, 14)	53 (49, 56)	34 (32, 37)	18 (9, 30)	8 (6, 11)
Not checked	88 (86, 90)	47 (44, 51)	66 (63, 68)	82 (70, 91)	92 (89, 94)

Equipment

Estimated percentage (lower bound, upper bound)					
Response	Total	Small hub	Non-hub	Non-primary commercial service	General aviation/ reliever
Checked	22 (19, 25)	10 (4, 21)[a]	35 (33, 38)	30 (19, 43)[a]	21 (18, 25)
Not checked	78 (75, 81)	90 (79, 96)[a]	65 (62, 67)	70 (57, 81)[a]	79 (75, 82)

B. If yes, in what ways did the CARES Act financial assistance and its implementation work well in supporting your airport?

Identified relief measures	Number of responses
Budget solvency (Relates to financial aspect of CARES. Responses may include combatting revenue loss, paying bills, debt covenant requirements, "stay in the black," meeting payroll, etc.)	268
Maintain level of service and/or operations (Relates to CARES Act impact on airport operations. Responses may include kept doors open, rates and charges, maintenance projects, services/operations.)	235
Avoid layoffs (Relates to impact of CARES on airport employees. Responses include avoiding layoffs and/or furloughs, allowing employees to keep jobs, and impact on staffing.)	87
Support projects (Responses include comments that relate to infrastructure projects, 100% match.)	74
CARES Act was well distributed (Relates to how the process was implemented. Responses include comments that relate to the process being easy, expedited, and flexible.)	77

Note: The above results are based on a content analysis of written responses. A total of 594 respondents provided a valid, written response to this question. Respondents may have mentioned more than one measure taken, therefore responses do not add up to 100 percent.

Appendix III: Staff Acknowledgments

In addition to the contact named above, Amy Abramowitz, Paul Aussendorf, Melissa Bodeau, Kim Bohnet, Jon Carver (Assistant Director), Gail Marnik, Josh Ormond, Justin Reed (Analyst-in-Charge), Gretchen Snoey, Larry Thomas, Elizabeth Wood, Sirin Yaemsiri, and April Yeaney made key contributions to this report.

Chapter 2

COVID-19: TSA Could Better Monitor Its Efforts to Reduce Infectious Disease Spread at Checkpoints*

United States Government Accountability Office

Why GAO Did This Study

Within TSA, approximately 46,000 TSOs stationed across the nation's commercial airports perform screening and other activities that often require close interaction with passengers. As a result, both passengers and TSOs may be at an increased risk of infection during pandemics such as COVID-19.

The CARES Act included a provision for GAO to conduct monitoring and oversight of the federal government's response to the COVID-19 pandemic. This report identifies 1) what steps TSA has taken to reduce the spread of COVID-19 at passenger screening checkpoints; and 2) how TSA is monitoring TSOs' implementation of amended safety and screening procedures, among other objectives.

GAO analyzed TSA data on TSOs' use of paid leave, reviewed documentation on policies and procedures, and interviewed TSA officials at headquarters and eight U.S. airports. We selected these airports to reflect diversity in the number of COVID-19 cases among TSOs, airport size, and geographic region. In addition, for six of these airports, GAO reviewed closed circuit television footage to observe how TSOs were implementing COVID-19 procedural changes.

---

* This is an edited, reformatted and augmented version of United States Government Accountability Office, Publication No. GAO-21-364, dated June 2021.

In: The Aviation Industry and COVID-19
Editor: Stefan Schneider
ISBN: 978-1-68507-712-9

What GAO Recommends

GAO is recommending that TSA 1) take steps to strengthen monitoring of measures to reduce the spread of infectious diseases at passenger screening checkpoints and 2) analyze available data to identify patterns of success and failure in implementing COVID-19 measures across airports nationwide. TSA concurred with our recommendations.

What GAO Found

To reduce the spread of COVID-19 at passenger checkpoints, Transportation Security Administration (TSA) officials issued amended safety measures to require that Transportation Security Officers (TSOs) use surgical masks and face shields, change gloves after pat-downs, and physically distance themselves from coworkers and passengers as practicable. TSA also adjusted some screening procedures, such as asking passengers to remove more items from carry-on baggage to reduce the potential for alarms that require bag searches. In addition, TSA modified the use of certain checkpoint screening technologies, and granted TSOs additional paid leave. In January 2021, TSA began an employee vaccination program, and is in the process of vaccinating TSA employees, including TSOs.

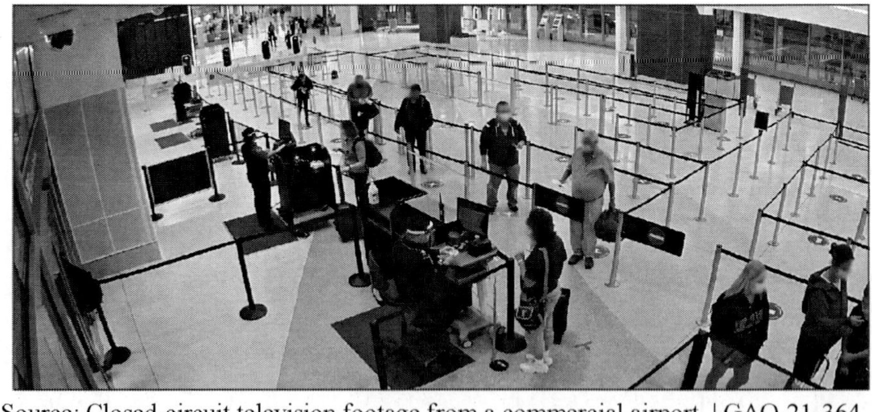

Source: Closed-circuit television footage from a commercial airport. | GAO-21-364.

Transportation Security Officers (TSO) and Passengers at an Airport Screening Checkpoint during the COVID-19 Pandemic.

TSA's monitoring and analysis of its measures to reduce the spread of COVID-19 is limited. For example, supervisors' operational checklists do not specifically include the revised COVID-19 procedures, and the data that TSO monitors collect (e.g., on whether TSOs are properly wearing masks or changing gloves) reflect implementation at a point in time rather than throughout a shift. Conducting more complete monitoring would help TSA ensure that its TSOs are properly implementing COVID-19 proccdures. In addition, TSA field leadership analyzes available monitoring data for different subsets of airports to understand how COVID-19 procedures are being implemented. However, TSA headquarters officials said they had no plans at the time of our review to analyze this data across all airports nationwide to identify common implementation problems, such as incorrectly wearing face shields and challenges with maintaining physical distance. Analyzing monitoring data across all airports would help TSA identify and address any system-wide deficiencies in implementing COVID-19 procedures, so that it may better protect its workforce and the traveling public.

Abbreviations

CCTV	closed circuit television
CDC	Centers for Disease Control and Prevention
COVID-19	Coronavirus Disease 2019
DHS	Department of Homeland Security
FSD	Federal Security Director
ICM	infection control monitor
OSHA	Occupational Safety and Health Administration
PPE	personal protective equipment
R&D	research and development
S&T	DHS Science and Technology Directorate
TSA	Transportation Security Administration
TSO	Transportation Security Officer

June 14, 2021
Congressional Committees

Since the outbreak of the Coronavirus Disease 2019 (COVID-19), approximately 46,000 Transportation Security Officers (TSO) employed by the Transportation Security Administration (TSA) have continued to perform tasks such as screening passengers at checkpoints, which may put them and the traveling public at increased risk of infection.[1] COVID-19 has had catastrophic impacts in the U.S. As of April 24, 2021, there were more than 31.8 million cumulative reported U.S. cases, and about 556,000 reported deaths, according to the Centers for Disease Control and Prevention (CDC).[2]

TSA—the primary federal agency responsible for securing passenger air travel—also seeks to ensure the health and safety of TSOs stationed across the nation's commercial airports.[3] Early in the pandemic, the federal government, in conjunction with state and local leaders, put in place interventions aimed at slowing the rate of infections. These interventions included travel restrictions, stay-at-home orders, and physical-distancing guidelines recommending that people remain 6 feet apart in public spaces. However, U.S. workers in certain sectors with mission-critical roles—such as TSOs—could not be fully protected by these interventions because their job duties must be performed in person. Therefore, throughout the pandemic, TSA has had responsibility for identifying and implementing strategies to prevent TSOs from contracting or spreading COVID-19 while they continue to screen passengers.

The CARES Act—signed in March 2020—includes a provision for us to conduct monitoring and oversight of the federal government's efforts to prepare for, respond to, and recover from the COVID-19 pandemic.[4] In addition, we were asked to examine TSA's efforts to reduce human-to- human

---

[1] The number of TSOs in March 2020 was more than 50,000. That number fell over the course of the pandemic, and by January 31, 2021, there were approximately 46,000 TSOs.

[2] Data on COVID-19 cases in the U.S. are based on aggregate case reporting to the CDC and include probable and confirmed cases as reported by states and jurisdictions. CDC's National Center for Health Statistics COVID-19 death counts in the U.S. are based on provisional counts from death certificate data, which do not distinguish between laboratory-confirmed and probable COVID-19 deaths. Provisional counts are incomplete due to an average delay of 2 weeks (a range of 1–8 weeks or longer) for death certificate processing. The data were accessed on April 27, 2021. Data include deaths occurring from January 2020 through the week ending April 24, 2021.

[3] While TSA exercises more direct operational control over certain aspects of security, such as the screening of passengers and property, it generally has no operational role in securing other areas of airports, such as public areas, and works collaboratively with airport operators and other stakeholders to respond to any security incidents. Subject to TSA oversight, regulated entities—such as airport and aircraft operators—implement access control measures and, in conjunction with state or local law enforcement agencies, must be capable of responding to an incident at their airport—whether in an airport public area or within an area for which access is controlled (i.e., a security-restricted area).

[4] Pub. L. No. 116-136, § 19010, 134 Stat. 281, 579. We regularly issue government-wide reports on the federal response to COVID-19. For the latest report, see GAO, COVID-19: Sustained Federal Action Is Crucial as Pandemic Enters Its Second Year, GAO-21-387 (Washington, D.C.: Mar. 31, 2021). Our next government-wide report will be issued in July 2021 and will be available on GAO's website at https://www.gao.gov/coronavirus.

contact at airport passenger screening checkpoints in response to COVID-19. This report assesses the following objectives:

1. How many TSOs have been diagnosed with COVID-19?
2. To what extent has TSA taken steps to reduce the spread of COVID-19 at passenger screening checkpoints?
3. How is TSA monitoring TSOs' implementation of the amended safety and screening procedures intended to reduce the spread of COVID-19 at passenger screening checkpoints?
4. How has TSA coordinated with other stakeholders to share and obtain information on steps taken to reduce the spread of COVID-19 at passenger screening checkpoints, and what have been the results?

Our review focused on those changes that were relevant to TSA's TSO employees, processes, and procedures in use at passenger screening checkpoints for the roughly 440 commercial airports in the United States from January 2020 through January 2021.[5]

To address our first objective, we analyzed data received from TSA for the period March 1, 2020 through January 31, 2021 showing the percentage of confirmed positive COVID-19 cases among TSOs. We used this data to examine COVID-19 cases over time, as well as the distribution of cases across airports by security risk category and geographic region.[6] To assess the reliability of these data, we reviewed TSA documentation and electronically tested the data for missing information and obvious errors, among other steps. We found these data to be sufficiently reliable for describing the distribution of COVID-19 cases among TSOs at the nation's commercial airports.

To address our second objective, we reviewed key policies and procedures TSA enacted to reduce the spread of COVID-19. We reviewed Department of Homeland Security (DHS) and TSA documentation of 1) procedural changes enacted and any new tools and technologies employed at passenger screening

---

[5] For purposes of this report, a commercial airport is any airport in the United States that operates pursuant to a TSA-approved security program in accordance with 49 C.F.R. pt. 1542 and at which TSA performs or oversees the performance of screening services. Additionally, for the purposes of this report, the term TSO includes private sector screeners employed by companies contracted with TSA to provide screening services at airports participating in TSA's Screening Partnership Program. See 49 U.S.C. § 44920.

[6] TSA oversees security checkpoints at approximately 440 TSA-regulated airports nationwide. TSA classifies airports into one of five security risk categories (X, I, II, III, IV) based on various factors, such as the total number of takeoffs and landings annually, and other special security considerations. In general, category X airports have the highest number of passenger boardings and category IV airports have the fewest.

checkpoints; 2) guidance on the use of personal protective equipment (PPE), such as surgical masks and face shields; and 3) human capital policies and flexibilities, such as amended leave policies. We evaluated the extent to which these were consistent with federal guidance from DHS, TSA, the CDC, and the Occupational Safety and Health Administration (OSHA). We also reviewed TSA time and attendance data for its TSOs to understand the use of expanded leave and telework options. To assess the reliability of these data, we reviewed TSA documentation and electronically tested the data for missing information and obvious errors, among other steps. We found these data to be sufficiently reliable for describing TSO use of different leave and time flexibilities during the pandemic.

Also to address our second objective, we conducted 21 interviews with aviation stakeholders about their experience with TSA's guidance and other tools to reduce the spread of COVID-19. These stakeholders included TSA Federal Security Directors (FSDs) who are responsible for ensuring TSA policies and procedures are carried out locally at airports; airport operator officials; and TSO union representatives at a non- generalizable sample of eight out of approximately 440 commercial airports.[7] We chose airports to reflect variations in 1) number of confirmed cases of COVID-19 among TSOs (including two airports with very few COVID-19 cases); 2) airport category; and 3) geographic region.[8] In addition, we interviewed officials from two private companies that perform screening at airports within our sample as part of TSA's Screening Partnership Program, a TSA program that uses private sector screeners to perform screening activities at airports.[9] We also reviewed closed- circuit television (CCTV) footage from six of the sample airports to

[7] We did not interview officials from each group at all eight airports. Specifically, we interviewed eight FSDs, six airport operators, and TSO union officials representing TSOs at five of the airports.

[8] TSA organizes airports into a hub and spoke system. Hubs are generally the larger category X or I airports, and many hubs are associated with one or more spokes that are generally smaller category II, III, and IV airports. We chose some airports that had smaller spoke airports that had experienced cases of COVID-19 to obtain FSD perspectives about how smaller airports implemented procedural changes to reduce the spread of the disease. For example, one of our sample airports was Orlando International Airport (category X), and its FSD also discussed experiences from its spoke, Orlando Sanford (category II).

[9] Specifically, one of the private companies conducted screening at one of our sample airports, and the other conducted screening at a smaller spoke airport associated with one of our sample airports. In 2001, the Screening Partnership Program was established in federal law, originally as a pilot program and then on a permanent basis, to allow commercial airports to use TSA-approved qualified private-screening contractors to screen passengers and property. 49 U.S.C. § 44920. As of April 2021, contractors performed passenger and baggage screening services at 22 airports across the country.

observe TSOs implementing the amended safety and screening procedures.[10] While our interview results and footage from selected airports are not representative, they do provide important context and illustrative examples. For example, interviews provided important insight into field employees' views of how TSA leadership communicated policy and procedural changes and the challenges that TSA field employees and airport operators faced as they implemented these changes.

To address our third objective, we reviewed TSA internal and published plans to assess the implementation of checkpoint screening procedures to reduce the spread of COVID-19. For example, we reviewed the monitoring checklist provided to field employees, as well as associated training materials regarding its use. We also interviewed TSA headquarters officials about any challenges associated with monitoring the implementation and effectiveness of these procedures. As discussed above, we spoke with FSDs, airport operator officials, and union representatives from a non-generalizable sample of airports to understand any local airport monitoring efforts, among other topics. Also, we reviewed CCTV footage from six of our sample airports to observe how field staff were implementing the TSA-instituted changes to policies and procedures and any associated challenges. We assessed the extent to which TSA's monitoring efforts are consistent with TSA guidance and the Project Management Institute's *The Standard for Program Management.*[11] In addition, the information and communication component of internal controls was significant to this objective, along with its related principle that management should use quality information to achieve its objectives.[12] Specifically, we assessed the extent to which TSA's monitoring efforts reflected this principle. Although the results from our review of airport footage are not representative, they do provide important context and illustrative examples, such as allowing us to understand the utility of CCTV footage as a monitoring tool that TSA leadership could leverage.

To address our fourth objective, we reviewed TSA's efforts to share and obtain information with aviation stakeholders on any new policies, procedures, tools, and technologies to reduce the spread of COVID-19 that could be implemented at U.S. airports' passenger screening checkpoints.

---

[10] We requested and reviewed CCTV footage from the initial set of six airports we interviewed. These were the airports in our sample with the most TSO cases of COVID-19.

[11] Project Management Institute, Inc., *The Standard for Program Management*, Fourth Edition, 2017.

[12] GAO, *Standards for Internal Control in the Federal Government*, GAO-14-704G (Washington, D.C.: Sept. 2014).

Specifically, we spoke to 1) aviation industry groups, such as Airlines for America and Airports Council International; 2) TSA's federal partners, such as DHS's Science and Technology Directorate (S&T); 3) the non-generalizable sample of FSDs, airport operators, and union officials described previously; and 4) officials representing organizations that engage with TSA's international partners, such as the International Civil Aviation Organization, and a non-generalizable sample of four TSA Representatives who engage with foreign governments within their areas of responsibility.[13] See appendix I for more information about our objectives, scope, and methodology.

We conducted this performance audit from May 2020 to June 2021 in accordance with generally accepted government auditing standards. Those standards require that we plan and perform the audit to obtain sufficient, appropriate evidence to provide a reasonable basis for our findings and conclusions based on our audit objectives. We believe that the evidence obtained provides a reasonable basis for our findings and conclusions based on our audit objectives.

Background

Impact of COVID-19 on Passenger Domestic Air Travel

Domestic passenger air travel decreased significantly in response to COVID-19, with a nearly 96 percent drop at its lowest point. Since April 2020, passenger volumes have been generally increasing, but remain about 65 percent below the volume one year ago, as of January 2021 (see Figure 1).

---

[13] Airlines for America is a trade association that works with member airlines, labor, Congress, and other groups to improve the aviation industry. Airports Council International advocates for policies and provides services for more than 300 local, regional, and state commercial airport owners and operators in the United States and Canada. The International Civil Aviation Organization is an organization that is funded and directed by 193 national governments to support their diplomacy and cooperation in air transport. Transportation Security Administration Representatives are TSA officials who are posted at US embassies and consulates abroad. They serve as TSA's interlocutors to foreign governments and advisors to Ambassadors and Chiefs of Mission on aviation security issues. They engage with counterparts, including foreign airports, and facilitate information exchange and dialogue.

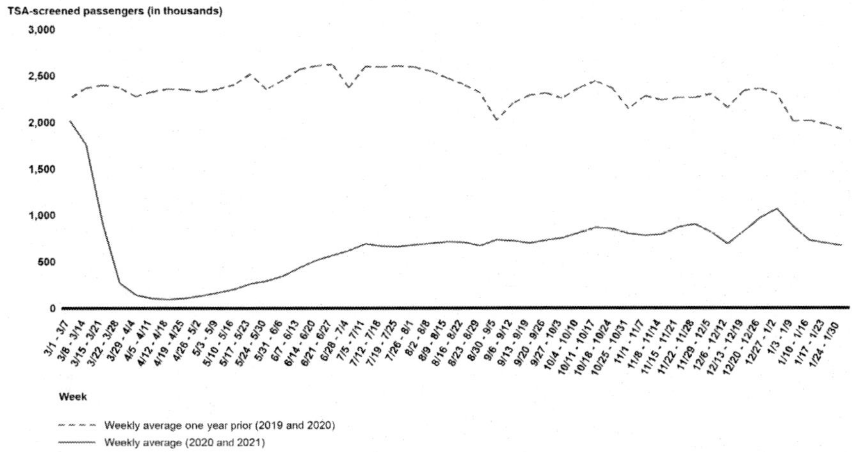

Source: GAO analysis of TSA data. | GAO-21-364.

Note: These data show the 7-day weekly average number of passengers screened by TSA. Data show passenger throughput in the current year (2020 and 2021) versus the year prior (2019 and 2020). Data for previous year (dotted line) were adjusted to match data for current year (solid line), so that all data shown reflect weekly data groupings of Sundays through Saturdays.

Figure 1. Transportation Security Administration (TSA) Weekly Average Airport Passenger Screening Checkpoint Throughput, March 2019 through January 2020 and March 2020 through January 2021.

TSA Roles and Responsibilities for Passenger Screening at Checkpoints

TSA Management of Checkpoints

TSA oversees security checkpoints at approximately 440 commercial airports nationwide, with its national operations divided into seven geographic regions across the country (see Figure 2).[14] TSA classifies airports into one of five security risk categories (X, I, II, III, IV) based on various factors, such as the total number of takeoffs and landings annually, and other special security considerations. In general, category X airports have the highest number of passenger boardings and category IV airports have the fewest. To ensure its policies and procedures are implemented locally at airports, TSA employs

[14] In March 2021, TSA officials told us that TSA had recently revised its field structure by reducing its geographic regions from seven to five. For the purposes of this report, we use the previous seven-region structure since that is how TSA provided data to us.

FSDs. Typically, TSA locates FSDs at larger (category X or I) airports, some of which also serve as hubs for smaller airports (categories II through IV) within a geographic area. These smaller airports are considered spokes of the larger hub airport. In such cases, FSDs are responsible for ensuring that TSA policies and procedures are carried out at both the larger hub and smaller spoke airports.

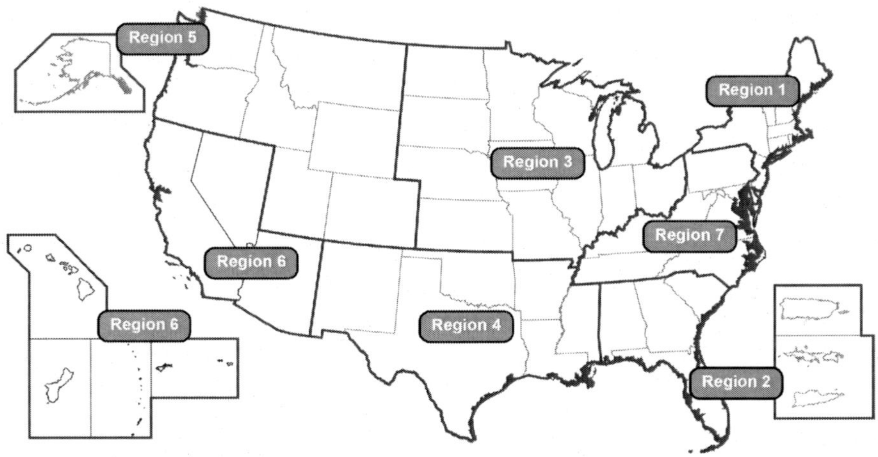

Source: GAO presentation of TSA information. | GAO-21-364.

Note: In March 2021, TSA officials told us that TSA had recently revised its field structure by reducing its geographic regions from seven to five. In the new structure, TSA combined regions 2 and 7. It also divided some states from region 5 and 3 across other regions, moving Washington, Oregon, and Idaho to region 6, and Montana, Wyoming, Colorado, Utah, and the Dakotas to region 4. For the purposes of this report, we use the previous seven-region structure since that is how TSA provided data to us.

Figure 2. Transportation Security Administration (TSA) Geographic Regions.

Checkpoint Screening Operations

The checkpoint screening process, as set forth in TSA's procedures, is intended to deter and prevent passengers from carrying any unauthorized or prohibited items into the airport's sterile area and on board an aircraft.[15] The screening process, as performed by TSOs, involves a variety of duties, including checking travel documentation for authenticity, as well as screening

[15] Sterile areas are security-restricted areas that, in general, provide passengers access to boarding an aircraft and to which TSA controls access through the screening of persons and property.

and (in some cases) searching passengers and their carry-on baggage for items prohibited on aircraft.

The checkpoint screening process begins when passengers enter the airport terminal security checkpoint and provide TSOs working as travel document checkers their boarding passes and identification for review. TSOs are to examine and scan boarding passes and identification documents to determine they are authentic and represent the passenger who is in front of them. To assist travel document checkers, TSA is in the process of deploying credential authentication technology at checkpoint entrances nationwide. The technology allows TSOs to scan passenger identification documents (such as a driver's license or passport) to confirm the authenticity of these documents and to help verify a passenger's identity.

After scanning and reviewing a passenger's boarding pass, TSOs serving as travel document checkers are to direct passengers to designated areas for standard, enhanced, or expedited screening. Before this screening takes place, TSOs serving as divestiture officers assist passengers with removing items from their persons (such as shoes) and within carry-on luggage and placing these items into bins. Most passengers receive standard screening. This typically includes being screened by advanced imaging technology, which identifies objects concealed on the person, and using X-ray equipment to screen the passenger's accessible property.[16] In the event that any of these screening devices identify a potential item of concern, TSOs are to take additional security measures as part of the alarm resolution process. These measures may include pat-downs or explosives trace detection searches, which involve using a device to detect explosive particles.[17]

---

[16] When advanced imaging technology is not available, TSA uses walk-through metal detectors. Advanced imaging technology provides additional capability compared to walk- through metal detectors to identify prohibited items on a passenger.

[17] *Enhanced screening* is generally required for passengers TSA identifies as high risk, such as those that have been matched to federal government lists of known or suspected terrorists. Enhanced screening involves the same procedures applied during a typical standard screening experience, as well as a pat-down and an explosives trace detection search or physical search of the interior of the passenger's accessible property, electronics, and footwear. *Expedited screening* is allowed for passengers TSA believes to be low risk. One group of passengers who routinely receive expedited screening are those enrolled in TSA's Pre✓®—a program through which individuals vetted and approved by TSA are eligible for this level of screening. Expedited screening includes walk-through metal detector screening and X-ray screening of the passenger's accessible property, and passengers do not have to remove their belts, shoes, or light outerwear.

Prior to the pandemic, TSOs were required to wear gloves for some activities, such as passenger pat-downs or searches of personal property.

Pandemic Guidance

TSA's ongoing response to the COVID-19 pandemic has been informed by internal and external pandemic-related guidance, including guidance from TSA, DHS, CDC, and OSHA.

TSA Pandemic-Related Base Plan

TSA has a plan to identify required management activities in the event of a pandemic. In 2017, as part of its Incident Management Framework, TSA issued its *Chemical/Biological and Pandemic Base Plan* (base plan).[18] The document includes requirements to conduct risk assessments, guidance on possible policy and procedure changes (such as leave flexibilities and changes to passenger processing) in response to a pandemic, provision for supplies and equipment (such as PPE), and other activities TSA should implement to limit the spread of a virus during a pandemic.[19]

CDC Guidance

The CDC, within the Department of Health and Human Services, has a mission to protect Americans from health, safety, and security threats, both foreign and in the U.S. In response to the COVID-19 pandemic, the CDC created a website for airports and their workers that contains links to guidance on limiting the spread of COVID-19.[20]

OSHA Guidance

OSHA, within the Department of Labor, helps ensure safe and healthful working conditions for working men and women by setting and enforcing standards and providing training, outreach, education and assistance. OSHA

---

[18] Transportation Security Administration Incident Management Framework, *Chemical/ Biological and Pandemic Base Plan*, July 2017.

[19] TSA developed its plan in response to requirements in the DHS *2016 Pandemic and Emerging Infectious Diseases Workforce Protection Plan*. Specifically, among other things, the DHS plan required that component agencies develop a pandemic response plan that contained specific elements to assist the component in protecting its workforce during a pandemic.

[20] For example, the website includes links to *Interim Guidance for Businesses and Employers Responding to Coronavirus Disease 2019 (COVID-19)*. See https://www.cdc.gov/ coronavirus/2019-ncov/community/worker-safety-support/airports.html.

has provided general guidance (Preparing the Workplace for COVID-19) and more specific COVID-19 guidance (Border Security and Transportation Security Workers and Employers).[21] These publications provide recommendations for cleaning and disinfecting the workplace and the need for PPE for different occupations based on the risk to the employee.

TSA Reported 5,456 COVID-19 Cases among TSOs from March 2020 through January 2021

Between March 1, 2020 and January 31, 2021, TSA reported that 5,456 out of approximately 48,000 TSOs (more than 11 percent) were diagnosed with COVID-19. TSA cannot confirm whether TSOs contracted COVID-19 while at work, because TSA's contact tracing process does not consider TSO activities and contacts outside of work.[22] Moreover, TSA does not provide access to testing for its employees. However, TSA does require local TSA management to report confirmed cases of COVID-19 in their workforce.[23] TSO infections increased as nationwide cases increased, and generally, the peaks in newly reported COVID-19 cases among TSOs are consistent with nationwide peaks in new cases on April 12, 2020, July 23, 2020, and January 11, 2021 (see Figure 3).

---

[21] See *Guidance on Preparing Workplaces for COVID-19*, OSHA 3990-03 2020, and https://www.osha.gov/coronavirus/control-prevention/border-protection-transportation-security, respectively.

[22] Upon receiving notification from an employee that their healthcare provider believes they have COVID-19, or the employee has received a positive test result, TSA staff are to alert local public health authorities, who may then conduct additional contact tracing.

[23] Specifically, local TSA management is required to report confirmed cases of COVID-19 in their workforce by entering incident information into the electronic WebEOC system. The system allows for two types of confirmation: 1) that the employee has signs and symptoms clinically compatible as identified by a healthcare provider, but the employee was not tested; or was tested and the result is pending; 2) that the employee received a laboratory-confirmed positive result. The system does not require management to indicate what type of testing was performed to determine the diagnosis. According to TSA guidance, employees must submit medical documentation within 14 days of COVID-19 diagnosis. Acceptable documentation must be from a local public health official or a healthcare provider who works in coordination with a public health official, and it must indicate when the employee was diagnosed as having COVID-19.

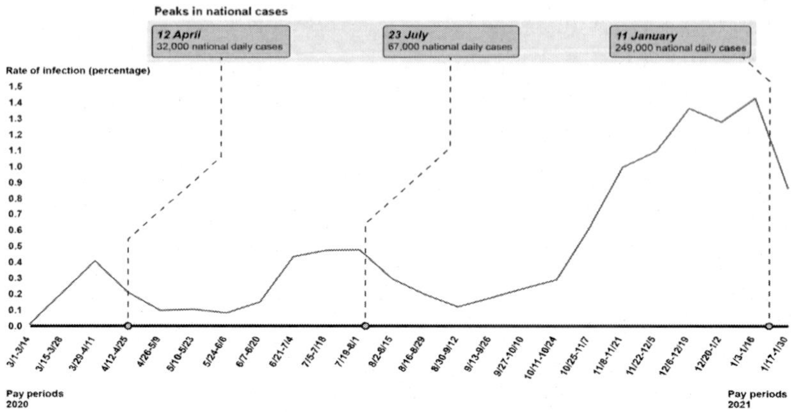

Source: GAO analysis of data from TSA and the Centers for Disease Control and Prevention (CDC). | GAO-21-364.

Note: This figure shows newly reported cases of COVID-19 reported to TSA by Transportation Security Officers (TSOs). It includes both (a) employees who have signs and symptoms clinically compatible as identified by a healthcare provider, but the employee was not tested, or was tested and the result is pending and (b) employees who received a laboratory-confirmed positive result. TSA cannot confirm whether TSOs contracted COVID-19 on the job. This graphic does not present data for January 31, 2021, as that was the first day of a new pay period. According to TSA data, there were 16 newly reported cases of COVID-19 on that day. National case lines represent the highest 7-day moving average of cases in the United States from March through May 2020, June through August 2020, and December 2020 through February 2021. CDC COVID-19 counts are subject to change due to delays or updates in reported data from states and territories. We calculated the relative difference between the average of new cases in the 14-day windows around the peaks in the spring of 2020, summer of 2020, and the winter of 2020-21, as of data available from the CDC Data Tracker on February 25, 2021.

Figure 3. Percentage of Transportation Security Administration (TSA) Transportation Security Officers Diagnosed with COVID-19 by Pay Period, March 1, 2020 through January 31, 2021, Compared to Peaks in Newly Reported Cases Nationwide.

A slightly higher percentage of TSOs stationed at category X airports were diagnosed with COVID-19 from March 2020 through January 2021, compared to TSOs at smaller airports. Specifically, 13.1 percent of TSOs working at category X airports were diagnosed with COVID-19. In comparison, between 8 and 10 percent of TSOs working at each of the other airport categories were diagnosed with COVID-19.[24] TSA officials stated that category X airports are typically located in dense urban areas, and this may contribute to the higher proportion of infections among workers at these airports.

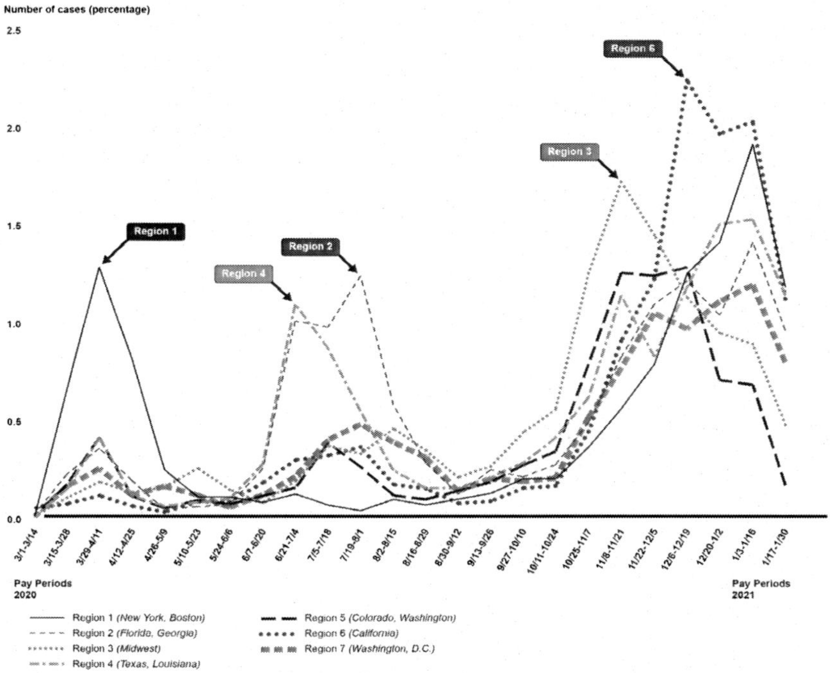

Source: GAO analysis of TSA data. | GAO-21-364.

Note: This figure shows newly reported cases of COVID-19. It includes both (a) employees who have signs and symptoms clinically compatible as identified by a healthcare provider, but the employee was not tested, or was tested and the result is pending and (b) employees who received a laboratory- confirmed positive result. TSA cannot confirm whether Transportation Security Officers contracted COVID-19 on the job. This graphic does not present data for January 31, 2021, as that was the first day of a new pay period. According to TSA data, there were a total of 16 newly reported cases of COVID-19 on that day.

Figure 4. Percentage of Transportation Security Officers Newly Diagnosed with COVID-19 by Transportation Security Administration (TSA) Geographic Region and Pay Period, March 1, 2020 through January 31, 2021.

[24] Specifically, category I airports had 9.8 percent of TSOs report cases of COVID-19, while category II had 8.9 percent, category III had 8.0 percent, and category IV had 9.6 percent.

According to our analysis, the region with the highest percentage of cases varied throughout the pandemic. Generally, the region that had the highest cases among TSOs in each time period was the same as the U.S. region that had the highest cases among adults overall. In the early weeks of the pandemic, the highest percentage of cases among TSOs occurred in the northeast region, where Boston and New York City area airports are located. In July and part of August, the highest number of cases occurred in the southeast region, where Atlanta and Florida airports are located. In December and part of January, the highest number of cases occurred in the west region, where California airports are located (see Figure 4).

TSA Has Taken Various Steps to Reduce the Spread of COVID-19

TSA's Initial Actions Included Conducting COVID-19 Risk Assessments and Implementing Its Pandemic Response Base Plan

Starting in January 2020, TSA began providing COVID-19-related guidance to TSOs and other TSA staff at airports and initiated its agency- wide response upon the declaration of a global pandemic 2 months later. For example, TSA began issuing employee bulletins, responses to frequently asked questions, and other COVID-19-related guidance to educate TSOs about prevention strategies throughout January, February, and early March 2020. According to TSA, this information was consistent with CDC guidance. TSA has continued to provide information and guidance to staff into 2021. In addition, according to TSA's base plan, TSA is to initiate formal management response activities (such as the formation of a management group to coordinate response activities) upon the declaration of a pandemic. Therefore, about a week before the World Health Organization declared COVID-19 a pandemic in March 2020, TSA began to implement the activities delineated within its base plan to oversee the development of workplace and administrative controls to reduce workforce illness and absenteeism due to COVID-19.

TSA implemented two key base plan activities early in the pandemic—assessing TSOs' risk of contracting COVID-19, and developing recommendations (based on OSHA and CDC guidance) to address it. Specifically, TSA's Office of Occupational Safety, Health, and Environment performed risk assessments (first in March 2020 and again in July 2020) to gauge the risk COVID-19 posed to TSA employees, including TSOs. According to TSA, the DHS Office of Human Capital determined these assessments were consistent with the DHS Workforce Protection Plan. According to DHS, the TSA plan is evaluated for consistency with CDC and OSHA guidance. The TSA risk assessments resulted in, among other things, recommendations for PPE. For example, TSA's March 2020 risk assessment recommended that TSOs wear nitrile gloves, but surgical mask and N95 respirator use were voluntary at the checkpoint. We discuss these and other PPE changes later in this report.

Other key activities TSA implemented from its base plan included reviewing existing policies and procedures to identify opportunities to reduce virus transmission. Specifically, these involved reviews of

- TSA's checkpoint procedures to identify opportunities to reduce transmission of COVID-19 at checkpoints, consistent with CDC and OSHA guidelines;
- TSA's human capital leave policies to determine how they might be used to reduce the spread of COVID-19 at the checkpoint; and
- TSA's acquisition and procurement policies. According to TSA, it streamlined opportunities to acquire necessary consumables, such as PPE, acrylic shield barriers (commonly known as plexiglass), and other tools TSA determined that passenger checkpoints needed to reduce the spread of COVID-19.

See appendix II for more information on TSA's management actions and procedural changes in response to the COVID-19 pandemic.

Throughout the Pandemic, TSA Revised its PPE Requirements, Screening Procedures, Use of Technologies, and Human Capital Policies

TSA made numerous changes to reduce the spread of COVID-19 at airport checkpoints. These included increasing its PPE requirements, revising screening procedures, modifying existing screening technology, and amending its human capital policies. FSDs, airport operators, union officials, and screening contractors we spoke with were generally pleased with the changes TSA had made. Some groups identified areas for improvement, such as the supply and quality of PPE, physical distancing requirements, and contact tracing, which TSA headquarters officials have been working to address. Figure 5 provides an overview of the key measures TSA has implemented at airport checkpoints in response to COVID-19.

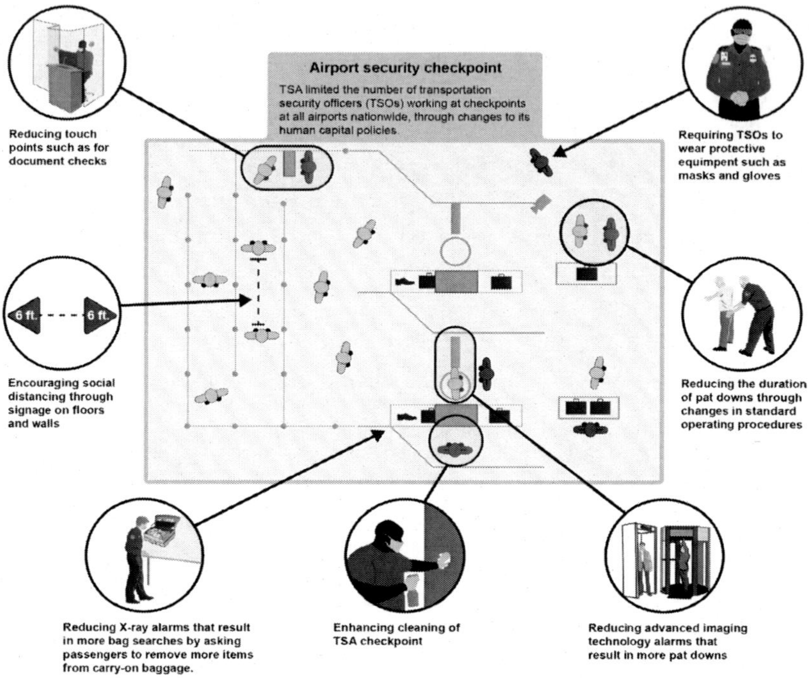

Source: GAO analysis of TSA information; Art Explosion (clip art). | GAO-21-364.

Note: TSA made changes to its screening process to limit the spread of COVID-19. That screening process begins when passengers enter the airport terminal security checkpoint and provide TSOs their boarding passes and identification for review. Screening typically includes passing through either a walk-through metal detector or advanced imaging technology machine (the latter of which identifies objects concealed on the person) and using X-ray equipment to screen the passenger's accessible property. In the event that any of these screening devices identify a potential item of concern, TSA conducts additional security measures, which may include pat-downs and bag searches.

Figure 5. Transportation Security Administration (TSA) Key Changes to Checkpoint Screening to Reduce the Spread of COVID-19.

Changes in PPE Requirements and Stakeholder Views

Since the beginning of the pandemic, TSA increased its TSO PPE allowances and requirements to ensure consistency with OSHA and CDC guidance. These ranged from allowing TSOs to use surgical masks and N95 respirators voluntarily in January and March 2020, respectively, to requiring that TSOs wear surgical masks and eye protection or face shields in May and July 2020, respectively.[25] Figure 6 shows the changes TSA implemented for TSO use of PPE in 2020.

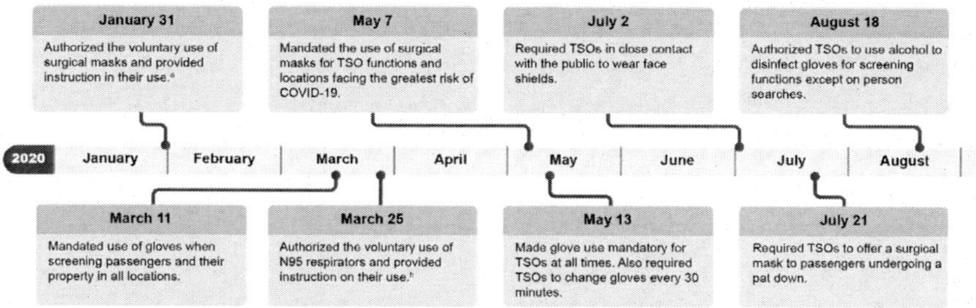

Source: GAO analysis of TSA information. | GAO-21-364.

[a]Surgical masks are loosely fitting masks that help block large particle droplets and splatter from reaching the wearer's nose and mouth and that reduce the exposure of others to the wearer's saliva and secretions.

[b]N95 respirators are tight fitting face pieces that require a proper seal, which forces inhaled air to be pulled through the respirator's filter material. They are used to filter smaller airborne contaminants.

Figure 6. Transportation Security Administration (TSA) Changes to Personal Protective Equipment Requirements for Transportation Security Officers (TSOs) in 2020.

In February 2021, TSA also began enforcing requirements for the use of masks among travelers related to an executive order to promote COVID- 19 safety at domestic airport passenger screening checkpoints.[26] The order, and subsequent Emergency Amendment by TSA, requires travelers aged 2 years

---

[25] By letter dated June 18, 2020, the U.S. Office of Special Counsel referred for investigation a whistleblower disclosure alleging that TSA did not take appropriate measures to protect its frontline workforce against the spread of the novel coronavirus (COVID-19), among other things. TSA's Investigations Division conducted an investigation into the allegations, and issued a report. As of March 2021, the U.S. Office of Special Counsel is reviewing the report.

[26] Executive Order, 13998, *Promoting COVID-19 Safety in Domestic and International Travel*, 86 Fed. Reg. 7205, (Jan. 26, 2021). The mask order, which was due to expire May 11, 2021, was extended by TSA Emergency Amendment until September 13, 2021. TSA Emergency Amendment 1546-21-01A (April 30, 2021).

or above to wear masks when they are in airports and while on passenger aircraft. According to TSA officials, TSOs who work as travel document checkers are to enforce this requirement at the entrance to the checkpoint.[27]

Stakeholder Views on Changes to PPE Requirements

FSDs, union officials, and screening contractors we spoke with were generally satisfied with PPE changes, but expressed concerns with the availability and quality of some PPE early in the pandemic. Specifically, FSDs from six of eight of our sample airports expressed concerns about the quality and availability of PPE, such as gloves, masks, and face shields, in the early months of the pandemic—a period when PPE availability throughout the U.S. was lacking. All FSDs who indicated there were problems with PPE early in the pandemic said the situation generally improved throughout 2020. We interviewed union officials representing screening staff at five of our sample airports. All five of them expressed concerns about PPE availability, and four said the situation with PPE had not improved at the time of our interviews in fall 2020.[28] Officials from one of the two Screening Partnership Program contractors we spoke to said they prevented PPE shortages at their airport by proactively procuring PPE beginning in January—well before the pandemic was declared.

TSA headquarters officials acknowledged that obtaining the needed supplies of PPE was challenging for TSA early in the pandemic, and said the agency has taken steps to address shortages. For example, starting in August 2020, to address potential glove shortages, TSA allowed TSOs to sanitize rather than change gloves in certain circumstances, such as when duties do not involve passenger pat-downs. Also in August 2020, according to TSA officials, TSA began to acquire a 60-day stockpile of PPE. Consequently, TSA officials explained that since mid-fall 2020, the agency typically has had a 2 to 3-month stockpile of PPE, in addition to a 60-day inventory of PPE sufficient to meet requirements for 100 percent of security screening operations.

---

[27] According to TSA, passengers who refuse to wear a mask will not be permitted to enter the screening process and will be denied entry to the secure area of the airport, which includes the terminal and gate area. Depending on the circumstances, those who refuse to wear a mask may be subject to a civil penalty for attempting to circumvent screening requirements, interfering with screening personnel, or a combination of those offenses. See Transportation Security Administration Mask Mandate Security Notice (Part Nine), February 1, 2021.

[28] Our sixth airport is part of TSA's Screening Partnership Program, and therefore does not have a TSO union representative.

Title and date of TSA guidance	Description of guidance
Guidance for Cleaning and Disinfection of TSA Workspaces *(March 2020)*	TSA's guidance provided guidelines for cleaning and disinfection of the checkpoint area and screening equipment. Among other things, the guidelines call for routine cleaning of frequently touched surfaces using 70 percent isopropyl alcohol and recommend cleaning products for both high-touch surfaces and all screening equipment.
Contact Tracing Guidance *(March 2020)*	TSA issued contact tracing guidance to be performed by TSA management for all cases of laboratory confirmed or suspected COVID-19 among Transportation Security Officers (TSO) and other TSA airport staff. The guidance requires that FSDs identify any staff who were in close contact with infected individuals, and to send these staff home on excused paid leave for 14 days.[a]
Coronavirus Disease Standard Operating Procedures *(May 2020)*	TSA'S COVID-19 standard operating procedures made changes to limit person-to-person contact during the screening procedures that TSOs must carry out at passenger checkpoints. Key changes include • requiring that TSO attempt to distance throughout the checkpoint from passengers and one another; • minimizing the number of screening activities that require TSOs to touch objects or passengers (touch points) by, for example, asking passengers to remove more items from carry-on baggage to reduce the potential for alarms that require bag searches; • reducing the duration of pat-downs through changes in standard operating procedure; • mandating TSOs use gloves at all times and change gloves after every pat-down; and • requiring the single use of explosives trace detection swabs.[b]
TSA Communicable Disease Response Playbook. (COVID-19 Playbook) *(June 2020)*	TSA officials developed the *COVID-19 Playbook* to identify and communicate to the field best practices for decreasing touch points and increasing physical distancing. Suggested practices include, among others • floor decals and signage to encourage physical distancing throughout the checkpoint; • the use of acrylic shield barriers at points throughout the checkpoint to protect TSOs who must interact closely with passengers (e.g., the travel document checker or the TSO assisting with divestment of personal belongings prior to the X-ray scan); and • designating a TSO to act as an Infection Control Monitor, to ensure that required procedures and suggested practices are being implemented. In addition, the *COVID-19 Playbook* aggregates all TSA COVID-19 policies, to effectively communicate requirements and suggested best practices to the field. For example, it includes a copy of the COVID-19 standard operating procedures.

Source: GAO analysis of TSA information. | GAO-21-364.

[a]The guidance when issued defined close contact as being within 6 feet for 10 minutes or more (cumulative) with the employee while the employee had any symptoms. The Centers for Disease Control and Prevention has since updated its close contact definition. According to this guidance as of March 2021, a close contact is someone who was within 2 meters of an infected person for at least 15 minutes within a 24-hour period starting from 2 days before illness onset (or, for asymptomatic cases 2 days prior to positive specimen collection) until the time the patient is isolated.

[b]Explosives trace detection technology uses a swab to test for the presence of explosive residue or vapors. TSA uses the technology on passengers and their belongings.

Figure 7. Transportation Security Administration (TSA) Guidance Issued in Response to COVID-19 in 2020.

Changes to Screening Processes and Stakeholder Views

In addition to PPE changes, TSA revised its checkpoint screening standard operating procedures and introduced new processes, such as contact tracing, and other best practices to address COVID-19.[29] To implement these changes, TSA issued new standard operating procedures for screening at checkpoints,

[29] TSA assessed all proposed changes to TSA's standard operating procedures to ensure none would have a negative impact on security. As a result of its assessment, it did not implement two of the proposed changes because it determined they would pose a significant risk to security. One of these changes involved TSOs' handling of passenger identification and another involved performing pat-downs.

new procedures for contact tracing when FSDs learn of confirmed or possible cases of COVID-19 among TSA staff or contract staff at airports, and other guidance on cleaning and best practices for protecting TSOs and passengers at the checkpoint. Figure 7 lists new procedures and guidance TSA issued in response to COVID-19.

Stakeholder Views on Changes to Screening Procedures

Most FSDs that we spoke with reflected positively on TSA's COVID-19-related procedures. Specifically, FSDs representing seven of the eight airports we contacted made positive comments about TSA's new COVID-19 procedures or TSA's efforts to support their implementation. For example, one FSD said TSA's procedures were timely and adequate. Another FSD said that TSA was in constant communication about the measures it was taking, which was reassuring.

FSDs and airport operators were less positive about implementing guidance and procedural changes as passenger volumes begin increasing from the lowest pandemic levels. Specifically, all eight FSDs and five of the six airport operators we spoke with said that physical distancing will be a challenge going forward once passenger volumes increase due to limited space at airports and the need to distance passengers throughout checkpoints. For example, the FSD and operator at one airport commented that physical distancing requirements at pre- pandemic passenger levels would result in lines that would stretch from the checkpoint into the airport parking lot.

In addition, FSDs expressed concerns about the potential for COVID-19 screening procedures to increase passenger wait times at checkpoints as passenger volumes increase, and TSA headquarters officials agreed. According to TSA, at the start of the pandemic, TSA headquarters officials encouraged FSDs in conference calls to ensure that checkpoint wait times should not exceed 10 minutes to limit passenger and TSO exposure to one another at the checkpoints. However, five of eight FSDs told us that if physical distancing requirements remain and passenger volumes continue increasing, a 10-minute wait time for passengers at screening checkpoints will not be possible. TSA's own research has confirmed these concerns. In summer and fall of 2020, TSA conducted two rounds of data collection activities to assess the impacts of COVID-19 procedures on checkpoint operations. At the time, passenger volume was 50 percent or less than it was the previous year. According to TSA, these assessments indicated a reduction in the rate of passenger throughput (i.e., passengers processed through checkpoints) of about 30 percent to more than 50 percent. TSA will conduct a third round of data collection beginning in April and continuing through August of 2021. In December 2020, TSA told us that to mitigate the impact of social distancing on passengers' queues and wait times, they directed FSDs to open checkpoint lanes at lower passenger throughput rates.[30]

Stakeholder Views on Contact Tracing and Cleaning

None of the FSDs we interviewed reported any difficulties implementing contact tracing and cleaning guidance. With respect to cleaning guidance, all FSDs reported that enhanced cleaning is performed by contractors or airport employees. In addition, two FSDs reported that additional cleaning is conducted when a positive COVID-19 case is confirmed, and one official representing a screening contractor at an airport staffed by private sector screeners said it created teams that went around the airport cleaning checkpoints continuously.[31]

With respect to contact tracing, six of the eight FSDs we spoke with discussed their efforts to conduct contact tracing to reduce the spread of the virus and keep employees safe.[32] FSDs from our sample airports reported using methods such as interviews and reviews of closed circuit television (CCTV) footage to identify close contacts among TSA employees while they were at work during the days leading up to their positive diagnosis.[33] In all cases, these FSDs reported conducting the contact tracing themselves, or in collaboration with local TSA or airport management or human resources staff. For example, the FSD at one airport reported creating a surge workforce of mission support and human resources staff, inspectors, terminal operators, and payroll employees to assist with contact tracing during a period when many staff at the airport had been diagnosed with the virus.

Some TSO union officials we interviewed reported that TSOs at their airports were confused by the contact tracing process. Specifically, we spoke with union officials at five airports, and officials from two of these airports

---

[30] According to TSA, it has traditionally staffed airports to avoid wait times in excess of 20 minutes but with the advent of COVID-19, it has been working to keep wait times to less than 10 minutes. To support this change, passenger throughput used in staffing models were reduced by 20 percent (150 passengers per lane reduced to 120 passengers per lane).

[31] It is TSA's policy after a COVID-19 case is confirmed to notify the airport authority or building management and to ensure the area is cleaned consistent with CDC and local health department guidance.

[32] The other two FSDs did not discuss contact tracing in response to our general question about their experiences implementing TSA's policies and procedures.

[33] The guidance advises FSDs to identify close contacts by looking at the employee's schedule and work location, and speaking with the employee about where he or she had been in the workplace (e.g., break room).

stated that some TSOs believed they had interacted with infected colleagues, but had not been identified for quarantine through the FSD's contact tracing.[34] Union officials at one of these airports told us that TSOs reported taking steps to get tested, despite not being identified through contact tracing. TSA has not pursued a program to facilitate testing for TSOs who believe they have been exposed to COVID-19, because, according to TSA, TSOs may use their healthcare provider and public health offices for testing. In addition, TSA implemented a vaccination program, which we discuss later in this report.[35]

Stakeholder Views on Other Guidance

All eight of the FSDs that we spoke to reported taking steps identified in TSA's *COVID-19 Playbook* to encourage distancing, such as by installing plexiglass, placing social distance markers on the floor, adding signage encouraging distancing, and removing seats from or otherwise reconfiguring employee break rooms. However, union officials representing TSOs at all five of our sample airports with TSOs reported concerns with management's implementation of *COVID-19 Playbook* practices. For example, union officials at one airport said that the decals on the floor had degraded over time due to heavy foot traffic, and have either been removed or were now illegible. In addition, union officials at three airports told us they see employee break rooms as too small to allow appropriate distancing, and that TSOs should be allowed to take breaks and meals at alternate locations.

Figure 8 shows passengers physical distancing at a TSA commercial airport checkpoint during the COVID-19 pandemic.

---

[34] The guidance, which aligns with guidance from the Centers for Disease Control and Prevention, was updated in April 2020 and defines close contact as being (1) within 6 feet for 10 minutes or more (cumulative) with the employee with laboratory-confirmed or suspected COVID-19 or (2) being directly coughed on in the face by the employee with laboratory-confirmed or suspected COVID-19. Additionally, the close contact must occur while the employee with laboratory-confirmed or suspected COVID-19 had any symptoms, or during the previous 48 hours before symptom onset. TSA requires its management (or screening contractors) at airports to report confirmed cases of COVID-19 in their workforce by entering incident information into the electronic WebEOC system.

[35] According to the DHS Chief Human Capital Office, DHS awarded a contract for the provision of COVID-19 testing in November 2020. The decision to facilitate testing is to be made by each DHS component (such as TSA) in conjunction with the component's medical officer, and as of March 2021, TSA has not participated in this program.

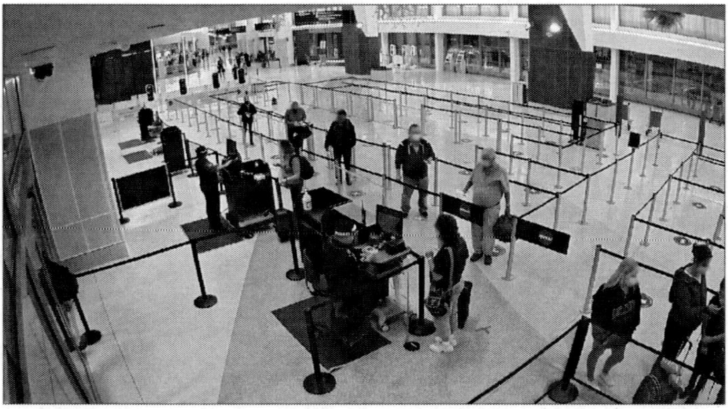

Source: Closed-circuit television footage from a commercial airport. | GAO-21-364.

Figure 8. Passengers Physical Distancing at a Transportation Security Administration (TSA) Commercial Airport Checkpoint, August 2020.

FSDs, union officials, and screener contractors from five of eight of our sample airports described practices implemented locally at their airports that could address some of the concerns union officials identified to us. For example, officials from two airports reported that TSOs were organized into teams, and sent on breaks together in order to minimize the number of coworkers that each would come in contact with throughout the workday. In another example, officials from one airport told us that employees are encouraged to social distance in empty terminals or to eat lunch outside rather than use the break room. Officials at two airports told us that to limit employees' exposure to others, TSOs were allowed to park closer to the airport terminals in which they work, so they would not have to ride airport shuttles.

According to TSA's *COVID-19 Playbook*, TSA is to periodically update this guidance as the agency develops new procedures. TSA headquarters officials responsible for updating the guidance told us they hold regular meetings with field health and safety officials and FSDs to share best practices and other locally implemented measures to prevent the spread of COVID-19 like the ones we heard about in our interviews with FSDs. Moreover, TSA has updated its *COVID-19 Playbook* three times since its release on June 20, 2020, to reflect its evolving understanding of COVID-19 and additional mitigation strategies being implemented by FSDs.

Changes to Existing Technologies

In addition to revising procedures, TSA also adjusted checkpoint technologies to reduce the spread of COVID-19. Specifically,

- To reduce TSO contact with passengers, TSA permitted FSDs to rotate credential authentication technology machines (used to validate passenger identification documents prior to entering the checkpoint) toward passengers to permit their self-scanning of documents. As of January 2021, TSA had deployed 1,053 credential authentication machines across 119 commercial airports. TSA plans to deploy 1,520 units by the end of calendar year 2021, starting with large airports (categories X and I).
- TSA made changes to the detection algorithms used by the advanced imaging technology machines to reduce the number of false alarms of passengers and baggage identified as needing additional screening.[36] This was intended to reduce the amount of close physical contact between passengers and TSOs, and limited the need for TSOs to touch passengers' personal belongings.
- For the walk-through metal detector, TSA directed TSOs to use a handheld metal detector to pinpoint alarms on passengers, so that they could conduct briefer, more targeted pat-downs to resolve alarms.

Figure 9 shows a TSA credential authentication technology machine deployed at a passenger screening checkpoint.

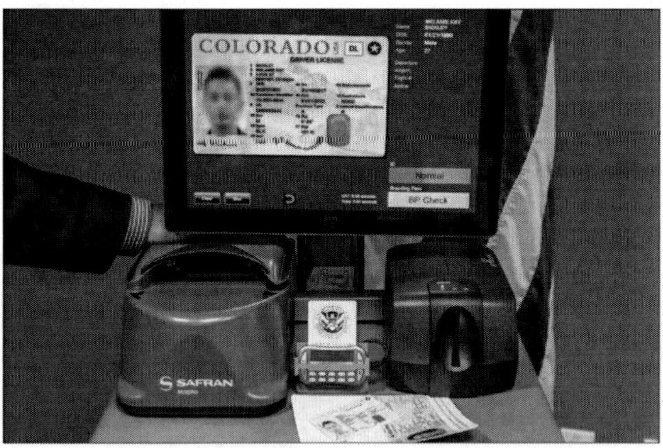

Source: Stephen Voss Photography. | GAO-21-364.

Figure 9. Transportation Security Administration (TSA) Credential Authentication Technology Machine Deployed at a Passenger Screening Checkpoint.

36 TSA assessed all proposed changes to TSA's standard operating procedures to ensure none would have a negative impact on security.

Changes in Human Capital Policies and Stakeholder Views

TSA also implemented new human capital policies to stem the spread of COVID-19. Beginning in March 2020, TSA began introducing new human capital policies that allowed TSA managers to grant TSA employees additional paid leave and to maximize telework when possible. With respect to TSOs, these policies allowed FSDs to grant telework or use weather and safety leave for TSOs who needed to quarantine due to close contact with someone with COVID-19, and to limit the number of TSOs at the checkpoint when screening activities were not needed due to decreased passenger volume.[37] In addition, TSA permitted TSOs to self- designate as high risk, which allowed these TSOs to be placed on extended weather and safety leave.[38]

Data show that FSDs used weather and safety leave more extensively during the pandemic to manage their TSOs at the checkpoint.[39] Specifically, TSA records indicate that FSDs permitted between 17,000 and 48,000 TSOs to use weather and safety leave per pay period from mid-March 2020 through January 30, 2021.[40] Over that period, FSDs used weather and safety leave the most from mid-March through early July 2020. Specifically, over that period, weather and safety leave accounted for between 16 and 62 percent of total time charges for TSOs. For example, at two of our sample airports, charges to weather and safety leave exceeded 70 percent of TSO time charges in at least one pay period. FSDs use of weather and safety leave decreased sharply

---

[37] An agency may approve weather and safety leave, a form of paid leave, if an employee (or a group of employees) is prevented from safely traveling to or performing work at an approved location. Employees may use weather and safety leave without the loss of leave to which they are otherwise entitled or a reduction in the pay of the employee or employees. TSA's COVID-19 human capital policies allowed FSDs to grant weather and safety leave due to reduced operational needs resulting from reduced passenger volume, among other things. In addition, TSA issued a Human Capital Advisory Memo on March 12, 2020 stating that an employee with a positive COVID-19 diagnosis would be placed on administrative leave/excused absence for a period not to exceed 14 calendar days.

[38] TSA's COVID-19 human capital policies define "high risk" as adults 65 and older and people with serious medical conditions like heart and lung disease, diabetes, high blood pressure, and compromised immune systems. Pregnant women and women who are breastfeeding are also considered at risk. Employees granted weather and safety leave are provided a notice that details the reason for the weather and safety leave.

[39] TSA also allowed TSOs to take weather and safety leave to attend to personal affairs related to the pandemic. TSA is not able report how much weather and safety leave has been used for each of the various reasons permitted by TSA's human capital policies. TSA issues a notice to employees identifying the reason for weather and safety leave— e.g., quarantine, reduced staffing requirements, etc.—but all use of weather and safety leave is coded the same in TSA's time and attendance system.

[40] These employee counts are for the number of employees using weather and safety leave each pay period. The same employee may use weather and safety leave in multiple pay periods.

between the pay period ending June 20 and the pay period ending July 4, falling from about 46 percent to 29 percent of hours charged. TSO charges to weather and safety leave continued to fall over the year to about 5 percent of hours charged by the end of December 2020, before rising to over 10 percent through January 2021 (see Figure 10).

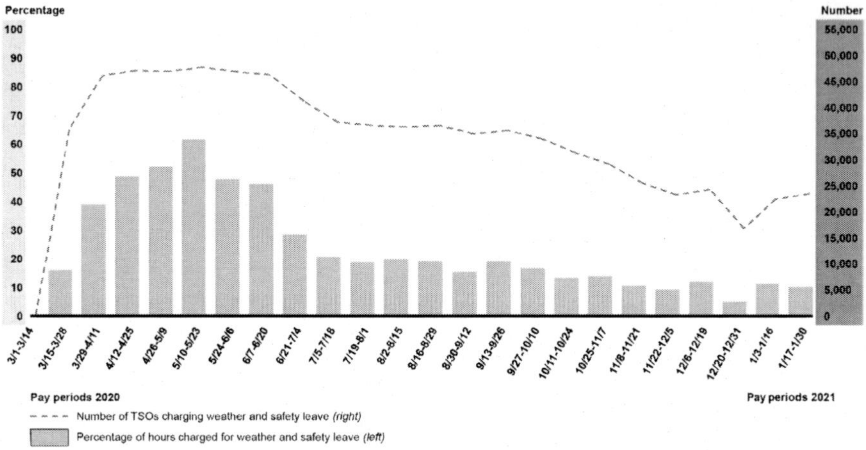

Source: GAO analysis of TSA data. | GAO-21-364.

Figure 10. Percent of Transportation Security Officer (TSO) Hours Charged to Weather and Safety Leave and the Number of TSOs Doing So, March 2020 through January 2021.

According to TSA, the use of weather and safety leave decreased for several reasons. First, passenger volume increased. TSA data show passenger volume increased six-fold from its low point on April 12 to September 30 (from fewer than 100,000 daily passengers nationwide to more than 600,000). In addition, TSA added an infection control monitor position, a new position using TSOs to monitor implementation of pandemic-related procedures and guidance, which added to staffing requirements.[41] Also, as previously discussed, in an effort to reduce passenger wait times, TSA asked FSDs to open additional checkpoint lanes, which required more staff. Finally, TSA eliminated the use of extended weather and safety leave for high risk TSOs on July 5, 2020, because, according to TSA officials, the agency was confident that its measures to reduce the spread of COVID-19 were able to mitigate exposure risks and made the workplace safer for all employees. TSA officials

[41] TSA's *COVID-19 Playbook* recommends at least one ICM for every 10 TSOs.

said that use of weather and safety leave dropped in late December and increased in January because staff took other leave around the end of year.

FSDs also increased their use of TSA's expanded telework flexibilities to address the pandemic, though they did not use it as extensively as weather and safety leave. TSA has a telework policy for its employees that states that TSOs are generally not allowed to telework due to the nature of the position and the requirement to be at an airport to screen passengers and baggage.[42] This limited FSDs' ability to use telework to manage TSOs during the pandemic. Specifically, TSA data show that fewer than 350 of TSA's approximately 48,000 TSOs used telework each pay period from mid-March 2020 through January 2021 (see Figure 11).[43]

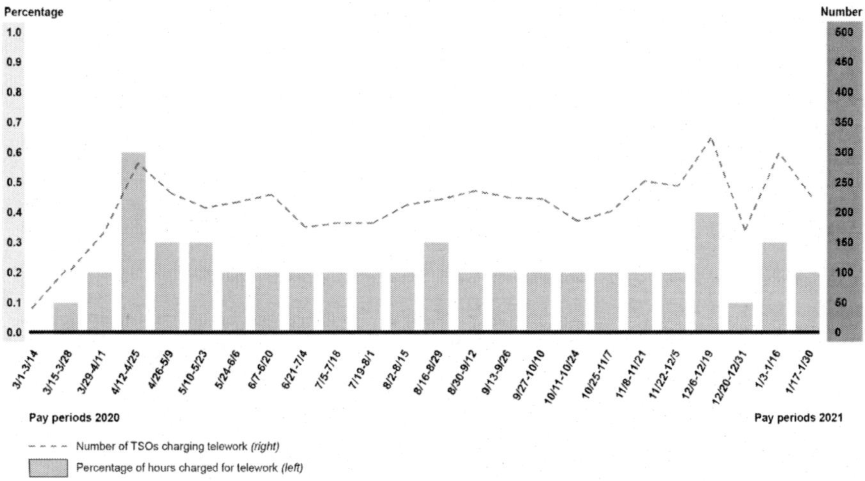

Source: GAO analysis of TSA data. | GAO-21-364.

Figure 11. Percent of Transportation Security Officer (TSO) Hours Charged to Telework and the Number of TSOs Teleworking, March 2020 through January 2021.

While FSDs used telework much less than weather and safety leave to manage TSOs, they still permitted TSOs to perform more telework during the pandemic than prior to it. For example, for the first pay period in March—prior to the introduction of TSA's pandemic flexibilities—39 TSOs charged time as telework. According to TSA headquarters officials, in order to allow TSOs to use telework, TSA created the Skills Advancement Initiative, which

[42] TSA Management Directive No. 1100.30.5 Telework Program.

[43] These employee counts are for the number of employees who teleworked each pay period. The same employee may telework in multiple pay periods.

placed 90 TSOs in developmental opportunities that could be performed while teleworking, lasting from 1 month up to 1 year, in support of TSA headquarters program offices. In addition, TSA officials also told us that TSA took part in a 90-day interagency agreement with the Small Business Administration that allowed 330 teleworking TSOs to support call center operations assisting small businesses with obtaining COVID-19 relief.

In addition to leave flexibilities, TSA issued new human capital policies in December 2020 and January 2021 to further assist and protect its workforce—specifically programs addressing worker's compensation and vaccinations for TSA employees.[44] In December 2020, TSA issued a new version of the COVID-19 human capital policy, which included information regarding workers' compensation. The updated policy directed employees on leave resulting from a positive COVID-19 test or a clinical diagnosis of COVID-19 who believe they may have contracted COVID-19 in the workplace to refer to TSA's workers' compensation management directive for more information about benefits that may be available to them under the Federal Employees' Compensation Act.[45] As of January 2021, 91 claims for workers' compensation have been filed by TSOs who believe they contracted COVID-19 on the job.[46]

Furthermore, TSA issued a new human capital policy in January 2021 announcing the establishment of a COVID-19 vaccination program in coordination with DHS and the Department of Veterans Affairs. This DHS program is ongoing and currently offers vaccinations at 22 Veterans Health Administration sites. As of April 20, 2021, almost 16,000 TSA employees had received their first dose of the vaccine, and more than 9,600 had received the second.

Stakeholder Views on Human Capital Policies

FSDs and TSO union officials we spoke with said they were generally pleased with the human capital policy flexibilities TSA offered in response to COVID-

[44] We did not solicit stakeholder views on these policies because they were issued after we conducted our interviews.

[45] TSA Management Directive 1100.00-6, *Workers' Compensation Program.* The Federal Employees' Compensation Act program assists federal civilian employees who have sustained work-related injuries or disease by providing appropriate monetary and medical benefits and help in returning to work.

[46] At the time of this review, 42 of the 91 claims had been accepted, 33 were still being adjudicated, and 1 was denied, among other outcomes, according to TSA officials.

19.[47] Specifically, all eight FSDs we spoke with were supportive of the use of weather and safety leave. Two of eight said it helped improve employee morale and another said it made physical distancing easier because fewer TSOs were at airports. However, union officials at four of five airports also said they believe FSDs at their airports should have allowed them to use weather and safety leave more, because, at the time we spoke with them, passenger volumes were still not approaching pre- pandemic levels. As discussed earlier in this report, TSA decreased its use of weather and safety leave in July 2020 because agency leadership was confident that the measures TSA put in place had mitigated exposure risks and made the workplace safer for all.

TSA's Monitoring and Analysis of Its Measures to Reduce the Spread of COVID- 19 Is Limited

TSA Conducts Limited Monitoring of TSO Implementation of COVID- 19 Measures

TSA monitors TSO implementation of procedures intended to reduce the spread of COVID-19 at the checkpoint through TSO supervisors and a new position called an infection control monitor (ICM)—a best practice recommended by TSA headquarters that FSDs may use to supplement monitoring conducted by TSO supervisors. However, TSA's monitoring efforts have been unsystematic and incomplete.

The Project Management Institute's *The Standard for Program Management* states that program quality control activities, such as quality reviews performed throughout the duration of a program, ensure that quality programs are implemented.[48] For example, outputs of quality reviews could include completed checklists and inspection reports, as well as measurement results. Moreover, they state that program management should ensure that proper risk policies and procedures are being followed throughout program delivery. Similarly, *Standards for Internal Control in the Federal Government* states that management should establish and operate activities to monitor the

---

[47] We interviewed TSO union officials at five of our eight sample airports, each of whom indicated they were pleased with TSA's use of human capital policies.

[48] *The Standard for Program Management*, Fourth Edition.

internal control system and management should use quality information to achieve its objectives.[49]

At individual commercial airports, TSO supervisors typically conduct monitoring of TSOs' implementation of required TSA safety procedures, including some measures that are important for reducing the spread of COVID-19. TSO supervisors are responsible for completing checklists at the beginning of each shift to document that the checkpoint is prepared to screen passengers. They also complete checklists at the end of each shift to document that all safety procedures were followed throughout the shift. However, these checklists do not include items specific to the revised COVID-19 safety procedures, and thus TSO supervisors are not systematically collecting data about their implementation as they do with other safety procedures. TSA headquarters officials said they ensure that TSO supervisors are monitoring COVID-19 and other safety procedures through regular calls with field officials, including FSDs, Designated Occupational Safety and Health Officials, and Collateral Duty Safety Officers. In these calls, TSA headquarters officials said they discuss the implementation of COVID-19 and other safety procedures and any concerns airport officials may have, based on their interactions with TSO supervisors at individual airports. However, because the TSO supervisors who conduct monitoring do not systematically record specific information within checklists about their observations on the extent to which TSOs are properly implementing COVID-19 procedures, headquarters officials have limited assurance that the information they hear on calls with FSDs and Designated Occupational Safety and Health Officials is complete.

To supplement monitoring by TSO supervisors, TSA established the ICM position in June 2020 for trained TSA employees at the airport; however, the position also does not provide TSA complete information on the implementation of COVID-19 procedures.[50] According to TSA, Lead TSOs typically perform ICM duties.[51] These duties include 1) providing TSA employees and passengers at the screening checkpoint with reminders about appropriate physical distancing and wearing of PPE, among other COVID-19 measures, and 2) ensuring that PPE, cleaning supplies, and staff are prepared

---

[49] GAO-14-704G.

[50] TSA guidance recommends TSA field leadership at the airport assign one ICM for every 10 TSA employees on duty.

[51] A Lead TSO leads a staff of TSOs, distributes and adjusts workload and tasks among employees, and oversees the security screening team on a daily basis. The Lead TSO is also to implement security procedures and provide coaching and guidance to TSOs in performing screening duties, among other things.

at the beginning of every shift. ICMs are also to complete a headquarters-provided checklist at the beginning of each shift that asks them to identify and document whether each of 16 procedures identified on the checklist is being implemented correctly, and if not, to list the corrective actions taken during the shift. ICMs are to then to submit completed checklist information into an electronic database each day for TSA headquarters review.

While the ICM position may be a helpful resource for airports attempting to ensure COVID-19 procedures are being implemented correctly, ICMs do not provide complete information on the extent to which COVID-19 procedures are being implemented correctly. This is because TSA headquarters does not require FSDs to assign ICMs and submit checklist data, and not all FSDs have done so for the airports they oversee.

Specifically, TSA officials said they created the ICM position as a best practice that FSDs may choose to implement if they have the necessary TSO resources and desire to do so. According to TSA data, TSA officials at about half of commercial airports have chosen to deploy ICMs and submit electronic checklist data as of December 31, 2020.[52]

Moreover, TSA headquarters officials who created the position said that when they did so they had expected ICMs to observe TSO behavior and provide ongoing feedback throughout their shifts. However, the ICM checklist instructs ICMs to fill it out at the beginning of their shift, before they have spent a meaningful amount of time observing whether TSOs are properly implementing ongoing COVID-19 procedures, such as correctly wearing PPE throughout the shift, changing gloves after every pat-down, or maintaining physical distance from coworkers and passengers. As a result, the checklist data that has been submitted is incomplete because it is unlikely to reflect the execution of procedures throughout a shift.

Using its current monitoring activities, TSA headquarters and FSDs are not in a position to understand the extent to which airports are experiencing challenges implementing COVID-19 procedures like the ones we observed. Specifically, we reviewed a selection of CCTV footage from a sample of six airports, and we observed examples of TSOs wearing PPE, such as surgical masks and face shields, both correctly and incorrectly at times throughout the time periods we reviewed. Specifically, we observed:

---

[52] TSA data indicate that 230 of 413 (56 percent) commercial airports with nonzero passenger throughput in December 2020 had submitted data from at least one completed ICM checklist as of the end of December 2020.

- TSOs serving as divestiture officers who were initially wearing their surgical mask properly, but would then pull them down and uncover their mouth in order to converse with a passenger that needed assistance.[53]
- TSOs serving at an advanced imaging technology machine wearing their face shield properly, but then lifting up the shield to talk with coworkers.
- TSOs who were not working near passengers initially, and thus not required to wear a face shield, but who then did not don their face shields when they approached passengers.

TSA headquarters officials said that they did not make the ICM position a requirement because they believed doing so would introduce an additional administrative burden on TSA staff in the field—e.g., time spent filling out the checklist and completing data entry. Officials said that even adding items to monitor COVID-19 procedures to the checkpoint opening and closing checklists that TSO supervisors complete would constitute an additional administrative burden. Officials also said they did not want to establish a monitoring process that was punitive at what was already a difficult time for TSOs.

However, TSA's efforts to collect monitoring information could focus on key activities, so that its monitoring resources target the most important procedures. For example, TSA could focus on correctly wearing PPE or social distancing by TSOs and passengers—and ensure information is collected on the continued performance of these activities throughout the shift. TSA could collect this information either through its existing monitoring activities (TSO supervisors or ICMs) or through another mechanism, without requiring punitive measures for TSOs who do not follow procedures.

Without systematically collecting complete information, TSA headquarters does not have full visibility on the extent to which TSOs at commercial airports are implementing key measures intended to reduce the spread of COVID-19 at the screening checkpoint. By taking steps to make its monitoring more systematic and the data collected more complete, TSA could help ensure its TSOs are doing so properly and also identify and address any recurring implementation problems.

---

[53] TSOs serving as divestiture officers assist passengers with divesting items from their property, such as carry-on luggage, shoes, and other removable items, into bins for X-ray screening prior to the advanced imaging technology or walk-through metal detector screening.

TSA Does Not Leverage Available Data to Identify the Extent TSOs Properly Implement COVID-19 Procedures across Airports

Through our review of CCTV footage at six of our sample airports, we found evidence of challenges implementing some COVID-19 policies and procedures across these six airports. However, TSA does not have plans to conduct system-wide analysis of the implementation of its COVID-19 procedures to determine the extent to which these and other challenges exist across all domestic commercial airports. For example,

- We observed examples across all six airports of TSOs not maintaining physical distance from coworkers and passengers, as required by TSA's standard operating procedure. For example, in some cases, a high number of passengers remained in the recomposure area to gather their belongings after screening, and this prevented TSOs from distancing from passengers. We also observed some examples where a queue of passengers would develop between the travel document checker and the advanced imaging technology machine and walk-through metal detectors. Consequently, we observed the TSOs stationed as travel document checkers did not have room to distance themselves. We also observed examples where TSOs would distance from one another while passengers were present, but they would congregate and socialize once there were no passengers to screen.
- With respect to plexiglass, we observed TSOs at all our sample airports that were meant to carry out duties from behind the protection of plexiglass do so incorrectly. For example, we observed divestiture officers and travel document checkers who chose to operate in front of or to the side of the plexiglass installed at their stations.
- Finally, we observed examples at all of our sample airports where TSOs did not use face shields and gloves properly. For example, one common occurrence across all our airports was that TSOs would lift their face shields like a visor so that it covered their foreheads rather than their eyes or face, which does not afford the additional protection TSA intended. We also observed TSOs at all our sample airports conduct multiple pat-downs of passengers without changing their gloves.

According to TSA's pandemic response base plan, after the pandemic is declared, TSA is to initiate a comprehensive after-action report process that reviews the effectiveness of its disease prevention workplace controls. As part of such a review, it is to identify patterns of successes and failures in steps taken in the field to address the pandemic. The results of the effort are to help TSA identify the response activities that it will include in future iterations of its pandemic response base plan. Furthermore, the Project Management Institute's *The Standard for Program Management* states program management should (1) ensure that proper risk policies and procedures are being followed throughout program delivery, and (2) use analysis to support program management decisions that respond to identified risks.[54] Similarly, *Standards for Internal Control in the Federal Government* states that management should establish and operate activities to monitor the internal control system and management should use quality information to achieve its objectives.[55]

TSA officials described a number of activities they have undertaken that they believe will provide information to help them assess trends in their implementation of COVID-19 procedures across airports. However, we found that these efforts were not comprehensive or did not involve a system-wide analysis of implementation data. For example, TSA headquarters officials said they have created a report based on the ICM data that FSDs at each hub airport and regional directors can produce and review. They said the report provides summary information based on ICM data for the hub (larger) airport and their associated spoke (smaller) airports. According to TSA headquarters officials, FSDs and regional directors can review these reports and provide them to headquarters leadership to help identify and communicate local challenges at an individual airport or at a hub airport and its spokes. While these reports may provide useful insight, especially at the local level, these reports include analysis for only a subset of airports.

TSA headquarters officials also described other outreach efforts that provide information on COVID-19 procedures; however, they do not involve an analysis of system-wide data. For example, they said headquarters has ongoing informal dialogues with FSDs and their staff about COVID-19 procedures. They also noted that in December 2020 they held a conference call with Designated Occupational Safety and Health Officials in the field to discuss questions and concerns about the ICM checklist. While such outreach may have provided TSA headquarters with useful information about field perspectives, they are, as officials described, informal, and do not involve

[54] *The Standard for Program Management*, Fourth Edition.

[55] GAO-14-704G.

analyzing data across airports. In addition, TSA officials said they conducted a survey of Designated Occupational Safety and Health Officials stationed at the 74 hub airports from December 21, 2020 through January 8, 2021. Officials from approximately half (49 percent) of these airports responded to the survey, according to TSA analysis, which included a few questions about these officials' experiences with the ICM position and their efforts to reduce the spread of COVID-19 at checkpoints. For example, the survey asked officials whether they believed the ICM program at their airport is effective and what their escalation process is for ICM checklist responses that require further action. While such a survey may have resulted in useful information, officials from half of airports responded and the results are not generalizable across all airports. Moreover, the questions included do not ask about TSOs' implementation of COVID-19 related procedures other than physical distancing in areas outside of public view. Therefore, the survey does not provide data to support a system-wide analysis of the implementation of COVID-19 procedures.

TSA routinely collects data on TSOs' performance of security screening requirements and analyzes this data to identify vulnerabilities and workforce training needs across airports. For example, TSA conducts regular covert testing at a selection of airport screening checkpoints, and testing teams report the results to TSA executive leadership to inform them about potential vulnerabilities to new and evolving threats.[56] Through our analysis, we identified data sources that would allow TSA to similarly assess, across all airports, the extent to which TSA is implementing procedures to reduce the spread of COVID-19. These data reflect first-hand observations of how TSOs are performing required procedures, and therefore could be used to support a system-wide analysis to identify trends in implementation. Specifically, these data sources include 1) completed ICM checklists, which, as we discussed earlier, TSA field staff at about half of the commercial airports regularly provide to TSA headquarters; 2) results of contact tracing, which FSDs or their delegates perform according to TSA guidance when a TSO reports laboratory-confirmed or suspected COVID-19; and 3) CCTV footage, which airport operators collect and make available to TSA upon request. For example,

[56] TSA selects airports where they run covert tests using a random process so that the results of their tests can be applied to screening activities at airports nationwide. The principles of inferential statistics require that samples be selected using a process that incorporates randomization, in order to make statements (i.e., to generalize) about a larger population based on analysis information collected from that sample.

- *ICM checklists.* TSA could use the data that ICMs are expected to submit daily to assess implementation trends, such as PPE usage and physical distancing across airports. Officials told us the agency does not have plans as of March 2021 to conduct analysis to identify trends across all airports, but that they could use ICM data to assess broader implementation trends if a larger number of airports submitted data. As discussed earlier, TSA does not have ICM data covering all commercial airports, but could leverage the data it has and supplement with other data, such as those described below, to ensure a more complete picture of implementation successes and challenges nationwide.
- *Contact tracing data.* TSA could also use information FSDs collect as part of their contact tracing procedures to better understand how well TSOs are practicing physical distancing. One FSD we spoke to reported tracking contact tracing data over time to measure the extent to which TSOs at one airport were maintaining physical distance from their coworkers while at work. Specifically, that FSD said they track the number of close contacts—as defined by the CDC—at work for each employee with suspected or laboratory-confirmed COVID-19. The FSD said that number, on average, has meaningfully declined since earlier in the pandemic. The steps the contact tracer is to perform, according to TSA guidance, allow FSDs to identify the number of coworkers who meet the CDC criteria of a close contact. Therefore, contact tracing results provide information on the extent to which TSOs are maintaining appropriate physical distance from coworkers while at work.
- *CCTV footage.* CCTV footage could also be used to assess TSOs' implementation of pandemic-related checkpoint screening procedures and identify examples of how TSOs are implementing procedures correctly. For instance, in our review of CCTV footage from six airports, we found many examples of TSOs correctly and incorrectly implementing some COVID-19-related procedures. Currently, FSDs review CCTV footage as part of their contact tracing process, so these officials are already familiar with what these video files can show regarding TSO interaction and other behaviors.

To use these data sources for a system-wide analysis, TSA could, for example, review CCTV data across a selection of airports, as we did, to directly observe examples of how TSOs are implementing COVID-19 screening procedures. TSA could then follow up by reviewing ICM checklist data to discover whether and how ICMs and field management responded to common deficiencies and develop additional training, guidance, or other mitigating interventions to help ensure correct nationwide implementation. Moreover, when its systemic analysis identifies successful implementation of procedures, TSA could likewise follow up to understand how airports supported these successes.

Conducting a system-wide analysis of monitoring and other implementation data to identify trends in implementing COVID-19 procedures would allow TSA to identify and address implementation challenges that are common across airports. Furthermore, all of this analysis could lead to meaningful lessons learned that might be applied against the spread of infectious diseases and future pandemics.

TSA HasCoordinated with Various Stakeholders to Identify Additional Ways to Reduce the Spread of COVID-19

TSA Used Existing Communication Channels with Various Stakeholders to Obtain and Share Information on Approaches to Reducing the Spread of COVID-19

TSA has used existing communication channels to obtain and share information on potentially useful approaches to reducing the spread of COVID-19 at airport checkpoints—including tools, technologies, processes, and ongoing research and development (R&D). Specifically, TSA headquarters has engaged with a variety of aviation stakeholders— including TSA field staff at domestic airports, representatives from domestic aviation industry groups, partners at international airports, and other federal partners.

TSA Field Staff

To obtain and share information on approaches to reduce the spread of COVID-19, TSA headquarters increased its outreach to FSDs and other TSA field staff to identify best practices and to encourage FSDs to implement guidance in a way that made sense locally. For example, in addition to the written guidance TSA headquarters provided to the field starting in January 2020, TSA shared information through town halls. Specifically, since March 2020, the TSA Administrator has held more than 20 virtual town hall meetings with TSA staff via live web stream from various airports and other TSA locations to provide updates on the agency's efforts to contain the spread of COVID-19.[57]

In addition to town hall meetings, in May 2020, TSA headquarters established an Advisory Panel composed of approximately 10 FSDs who meet at least biweekly to provide feedback on the implementation of new COVID-19-related procedures and guidance and share any innovative measures they had implemented to reduce the spread of the virus. This forum allowed, for example, an FSD in Michigan to share his airport's practice of rotating the credential authentication technology machine at the screening checkpoint toward passengers—a practice that the agency later included in its *COVID-19 Playbook* guidance.

Aviation Industry Groups

TSA regularly consults with its aviation industry partners on a range of issues, including the COVID-19 pandemic. These industry partners include TSA's Aviation Security Advisory Committee, as well as individual industry groups such as Airlines for America and the Airports Council International.[58] Representatives we spoke with from these groups reported a satisfactory level of communication with TSA management during the pandemic. For example, officials from Airlines for America reported TSA had been transparent with industry partners about both the measures they would implement to address the pandemic and the challenges to protecting their workforce.

Officials from these groups also reported that TSA management consistently engaged with them to identify best practices for limiting human-to-human contact throughout the aviation travel process and on new technologies to help reduce the spread of COVID-19. Cleaning and sanitization have been consistent areas of interest during conversations between TSA and these groups. For example, Airlines for America officials

---

57 TSA held these virtual town hall meetings from five airports (Boston Logan International Airport, Hartsfield-Jackson Atlanta International Airport, Chicago O'Hare International Airport, Newark Liberty International Airport, and Dallas-Fort Worth International Airport), the agency's headquarters, and the TSA Transportation Security Operations Center.

58 The Aviation Security Advisory Committee, which is composed of individuals representing private sector organizations affected by aviation security requirements, advises TSA leadership on aviation security matters, including the development and implementation of policies, programs, rulemaking, and security directives pertaining to aviation security. Airlines for America is a trade association that works with member airlines, labor, Congress, and other groups to improve the aviation industry. Airports Council International advocates for policies and provides services for more than 300 local, regional, and state commercial airport owners and operators in the United States and Canada.

reported that they have regular discussions with TSA about efforts to routinely clean areas around checkpoints and better sanitization processes for the bins used by passengers going through the security checkpoints.

International Aviation Stakeholders

According to TSA headquarters officials, they have exchanged information on approaches to reducing the spread of COVID-19 with international stakeholders throughout the pandemic. These efforts have included TSA Representatives who engage with foreign governments, and the agency's International and Interagency COVID-19 Working Group. According to TSA headquarters officials, TSA Representatives stationed abroad have provided information to internal stakeholders in charge of capability development within TSA's Office of Requirements and Capabilities Analysis on strategies to reduce the spread of COVID-19 that they have observed at the foreign airports within regions where they are posted. For example, one TSA Representative shared information about various technologies to clean airport surfaces with ultraviolet radiation in use at an airport within her region with officials from TSA's office of Requirements and Capabilities Analysis. According to the Representative, her airport's positive outcomes using ultraviolet radiation influenced TSA's decision to continue pursuing this technology at U.S. airports. Another TSA Representative provided information on the local airport authority's decision to increase the limit allowed for passenger hand sanitizer from 3.4 to 12 fluid ounces. This information helped TSA implement a similar change at domestic airports.

TSA Representatives abroad whom we interviewed also indicated that having pre-existing information-sharing agreements helped facilitate the exchange of information on COVID-19-related issues. According to TSA officials, the agency established these agreements to allow for the exchange of sensitive or classified information between aviation stakeholders abroad and government officials.[59] For example, one TSA Representative we interviewed said that having the information-sharing tools already in place allowed for faster exchange about countries' pandemic response plans and another emphasized that the agreements helped ensure that countries' security standards remained aligned.

In addition, TSA created the International and Interagency COVID-19 Working Group in May 2020 to monitor mitigation solutions under

[59] TSA headquarters officials noted, however, that much of the COVID-19-related information shared with foreign partners was not categorized as sensitive or classified.

development and other research by different foreign partners. According to TSA, this working group has conducted outreach with more than 20 foreign aviation sector partners to exchange COVID-19-related mitigation solutions and has documented similarities and differences among these solutions. For example, TSA found that most of its international partners are pursuing social distance queuing (e.g., floor decals and signage) as their main checkpoint design change. Conversely, TSA also noted that none of its international counterparts have chosen to adopt a safety officer position similar to its ICM position.[60] According to TSA, the information collected through these efforts is provided to internal TSA stakeholders to help prioritize R&D activities. In addition, TSA officials reported representing the U.S. Government in an international effort to develop high-level guidance for governments and industry to begin restarting international air transport and recovery from COVID-19.[61]

Federal Partners

TSA headquarters officials explained they have worked most closely with staff from the DHS Science and Technology directorate (S&T) to obtain information on COVID-19-related R&D, but they are also monitoring research by other federal entities that may be useful.[62] In the past, TSA has partnered with DHS S&T on researching new technologies to improve passenger screening at airport checkpoints. Officials from DHS S&T stated that they began discussions with TSA on specific COVID-19- related research projects for airport checkpoints in May 2020. In particular, DHS S&T officials said their long-standing partnership with TSA on R&D for other checkpoint technologies helped the two agencies negotiate research priorities that could be accomplished faster than other agencies that were less familiar with DHS S&T. For example, they said that DHS S&T was able to append quickly TSA-specific requests onto its existing COVID-19-related R&D. Consequently, TSA is coordinating with DHS S&T on several R&D projects related to

---

[60] TSA officials said that although none of the international partners it consulted have established the safety officer role within their airports, these partners continue to modify and evolve their COVID-19 mitigation strategies. TSA officials have noted that some of their international partners have expressed interest in TSA's requirements, training, and responsibilities for its ICM position.

[61] This guidance was developed under the auspices of the International Civil Aviation Organization, an organization that is funded and directed by 193 national governments to support their diplomacy and cooperation in air transport.

[62] Within DHS, S&T is responsible for coordinating and integrating R&D activities across the department. DHS components may also conduct R&D to support their respective missions.

reducing the spread of COVID-19 at the checkpoint, which we discuss later in this report.

In addition, DHS S&T officials told us that they have created a master question list regarding COVID-19 research that they have been updating since January 2020. The list is shared with DHS components including TSA and is derived from a range of sources (such as reports and articles found in scientific and technical journals) and serves as a repository for information on COVID-19-related R&D across the federal government.

TSA Is Pursuing Five R&D Initiatives and Has Fast-Tracked Planned Technology Upgrades

Since May 2020, TSA has partnered with DHS S&T on five R&D projects to limit the spread of COVID-19 at the checkpoint, and is also working to fast-track technology upgrades planned prior to the pandemic for technologies that may have the collateral benefit of limiting the spread of COVID-19 at checkpoints.

R&D Initiatives

TSA is coordinating with DHS S&T on five R&D efforts to reduce the spread of COVID-19 at the checkpoint for possible implementation (see Figure 12).

According to TSA officials, DHS S&T has provided preliminary results for four of the five measures and a final report for the fifth measure related to the effectiveness of TSA-approved cleaning solutions in disinfecting security checkpoints. These officials told us that they do not intend to delay moving these measures to the next phase of implementation if preliminary results support moving forward with additional pilot tests rather than waiting for the final reports from DHS S&T. For example, they are currently testing ultraviolet light bin disinfection in the field despite the final report not being complete, and officials are planning to utilize these tests to inform subsequent risk assessments for this technology.[63]

[63] TSA expects to receive results from the remaining four workflows from DHS S&T in late spring 2021.

	Requested Activities	Anticipated Impacts
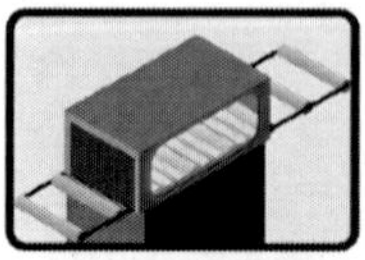	**Ultra Violet (UV) Light Bin Disinfection:** Assess the efficacy of alternative commercial UV lighting to eliminate the presence of COVID-19 on high-touch items used during checkpoint screening, such as bins to hold passengers' belongings during X-ray screening.	Integrate commercial germicidal UV light technology into passenger screening process to support bin decontamination.
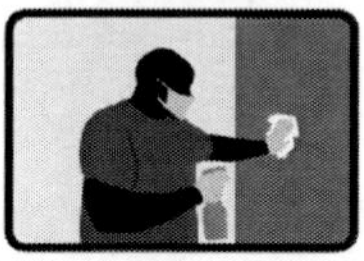	**Cleaning Solutions:** Assess efficacy of TSA's approved cleaning solutions to disinfect checkpoint surfaces. Research COVID-19 virus survivability across range of surface types and required contact times.	Identify whether various chemicals— including disinfectants available as commercial, off-the-shelf disinfectants— can be used to effectively meet checkpoint cleaning standards.
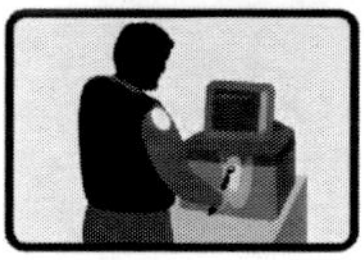	**Explosives Trace Detection (ETD)[b] Swabs:** Investigate the possibility of reutilizing ETD swabs based on the potential for the high temperatures ETDs generate during screening to eliminate the presence of the virus on sample media.	Determine the stability of the COVID-19 virus on ETD swabs and potentially eliminate the operational requirement to limit sampling of ETD swabs to a single use.
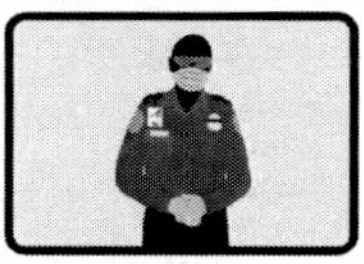	**Face Coverings:** Review alternative, cloth-based Transportation Security Officer (TSO) face coverings to assess COVID-19 survivability on cloth material, filtration efficiency, and side leakage.	Identify materials suitable for use in the procurement of face coverings to inform future personal protective equipment purchases for TSOs.
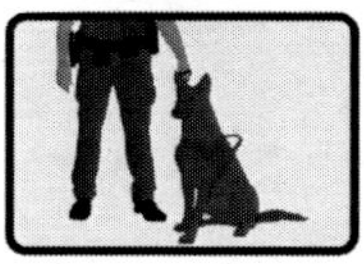	**Canine Studies:** Identify alternative canine training methods and aids to detect individuals with COVID-19 biomarker signatures and checkpoint surfaces contamination.	Possible use of canines to 1) identify COVID-19 positive passengers, and 2) validate that checkpoint surfaces are not contaminated with the COVID-19 virus.

Source: GAO analysis of TSA information. | GAO-21-364.

[a]In addition to these five research projects, TSA and DHS Science & Technology have collaborated on a sixth project related to Aircraft Airflow Modeling to characterize viral particle movement on airplanes. We did not include this study in our list of research and development projects because it does not address checkpoint operations.

[b]Explosives trace detection technology uses a swab to test for the presence of explosive particles. TSA uses the technology on passengers and their belongings if initial x-ray or advanced imaging technology identify a possible threat item. Per the new COVID-19 Standard Operating Procedures, TSOs are to change explosives trace detection swabs after each screening.

Figure 12. Transportation Security Administration (TSA) and Department of Homeland Security's Science and Technology Directorate Research and Development Initiatives to Reduce the Spread of COVID-19 at Screening Checkpoints.[a]

With regard to ultraviolet light technology, preliminary results showed that short-wave ultraviolet light proved effective at inactivating the virus on passenger screening bins.[64] TSA selected three ultraviolet light standalone bin disinfection systems from two unique vendors, and in March 2021, began pilot testing two of the three systems at airports (see Figure 13).[65] Additionally, TSA is also exploring integrated ultraviolet light systems that could be incorporated into pre-existing screening lane tray return systems (i.e., the trays travel back to the next passenger after security screening is completed). According to TSA officials, they have begun to evaluate the effectiveness of these integrated solutions and plan to pilot these systems to determine whether they can progress through an expedited acquisition review process.

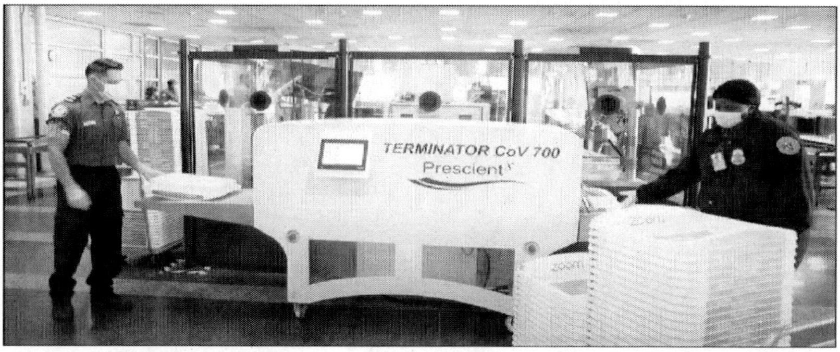

Source: TSA. | GAO-21-364.

Figure 13. Transportation Security Administration (TSA) Piloting Standalone Ultraviolet Light Bin Disinfection Systems.

In addition to the five DHS S&T R&D efforts, TSA is following, but not actively pursuing, a number of ongoing R&D efforts by other federal partners that may help reduce the spread of COVID-19 at checkpoints. Specifically, TSA has a list of approximately 40 COVID-19 R&D efforts that it is monitoring.[66] The list includes a number of R&D projects overseen by the Department of Energy's National Laboratories, including efforts to model virus transmission in closed spaces and rapid COVID-19 diagnostic tools. TSA officials also said the agency is following R&D being conducted by the

[64] The ultraviolet light spectrum can be broken down into three categories: short-wave, middle-wave, and long-wave. DHS S&T tested the effectiveness of short wave ultra violet light in decontaminating passenger screening bins and found this method to be effective at inactivating the COVID-19 virus.

[65] According to TSA, all three ultraviolet light solutions underwent safety evaluations to determine whether each system could efficiently kill the COVID-19 virus, as determined by DHS S&T and TSA. As a result of these tests, two of the three systems were chosen for live pilot testing at screening checkpoints.

[66] The list also includes a number of private sector R&D efforts as well.n.

Environmental Protection Agency to better understand efforts to characterize long-term antimicrobial pesticide products for use at high-touch areas.[67]

Planned Technology Upgrades

In addition to partnering on DHS S&T's R&D, TSA has also fast-tracked the planned implementation of technologies that have the potential to further reduce touch points at checkpoints. For example, TSA officials said that as of April 2021, there were 300 computed tomography (CT) systems deployed across 235 checkpoints and 4 labs.[68] According to TSA, CT has improved threat detection capabilities for carry-on baggage at security checkpoints, which further reduces touch points (i.e., the number of bag checks TSOs must perform) for TSOs (see Figure 14).[69]

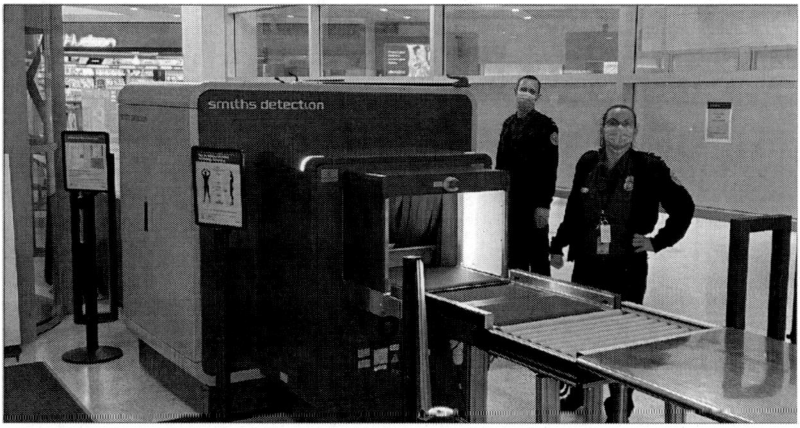

Source: Transportation Security Administration. | GAO-21-364.

Figure 14. Transportation Security Administration (TSA) Computed Tomography Checkpoint Screening Machine.

---

[67] This effort will characterize the product's effectiveness and durability based on time, physical contact, and degradation susceptibility to routine cleaning solutions.

[68] CT technology provides enhanced detection of threat items. TSA's current screening technology for carry-on bags uses two-dimensional images. The CT technology applies sophisticated algorithms for the detection of explosives and other threats by creating a 3-D image that can be viewed and rotated 360 degrees for a thorough analysis.

[69] According to TSA officials, TSA plans to increase deployment of these systems using competitive awards. The Checkpoint Property Screening System program released the first solicitation in November 2020, with an anticipated award for approximately 223 mid- size systems in the fourth quarter of fiscal year 2021 and deployment beginning in the first quarter of fiscal year 2022. According to TSA the planned procurement of these systems has since changed, and the program now intends on procuring approximately 242 mid- size systems.

TSA is also in the process of developing a new self-service credential authentication technology device equipped with a camera that compares a passenger's live facial image against the image from their identity document.[70] As of March 2021, TSA was pilot testing these machines.[71] According to TSA officials, these new models would be oriented toward passengers, who will be able to scan their own identification rather than physically handing it to a TSO. TSA officials believe that the credential authentication technology units would further reduce the risk of contracting COVID-19 at the checkpoint by limiting touch points and time spent in close proximity between potentially contagious passengers and TSOs.

Furthermore, TSA's efforts to obtain and share information on COVID-19 mitigation strategies have led to its decision not to pursue certain technologies. For example, TSA officials said the agency was not pursuing approximately 40 tools and strategies to limit COVID-19, ranging from tools to monitor passenger vital signs to mechanisms designed to filter information on social media. In addition, TSA abandoned temperature screenings at checkpoints for its TSO workforce and individual passengers, based on guidance jointly developed by DHS and the departments of Transportation and Health and Human Services. That guidance states that temperature screenings are unable to detect asymptomatic or pre-symptomatic people with COVID-19, those who are ill but who do not have fever, and those who have treated their fever with medication. Therefore, the guidance states temperature screenings should not be relied upon as a standalone public health measure.[72]

Conclusion

The COVID-19 pandemic has greatly impacted the demand for air travel and the people working in the air transportation industry. Thousands of TSA's

[70] As of December 2020, credential authentication machines deployed at checkpoints can validate that the identity document presented by the passenger is authentic, but do not have cameras. Only the units in the pilot program have cameras.

[71] According to TSA, formal field tests are being conducted with volunteer passengers at Ronald Reagan Washington National Airport, Phoenix Sky Harbor Airport, Indianapolis International Airport, and Miami International Airport to evaluate the system's performance across diverse operational environments and demographics to identify, understand, and mitigate variations in system performance. Following these field pilots, TSA plans to acquire additional units to conduct extended field pilots before making a final deployment decision.

[72] *Runway to Recovery: The United States Framework for Airlines and Airports to Mitigate the Public Health Risks of Coronavirus Guidance* Jointly issued by the U.S. Departments of Transportation, Homeland Security, and Health and Human Services, (July 2020).

staff, most of them TSOs who work at passenger checkpoints at airports across the country, have contracted COVID-19. In January 2020, when the U.S. experienced its first cases of the virus, TSA began coordinating its response to the pandemic and implementing an array of changes to reduce the spread of COVID-19 at airport checkpoints. These changes included 1) requiring TSOs to use personal protective equipment; 2) amending passenger screening procedures to reduce TSO exposure to potentially infected passengers and other new procedural guidance; 3) modifying existing screening technology; and 4) adding human capital flexibilities that reduced TSO exposure at the checkpoint.

It is important to the safety of TSA employees, passengers, and the function of the aviation sector that TSOs appropriately implement policies and procedures to limit the spread of COVID-19. TSA has processes to monitor the implementation of safety procedures, such as those intended to stem the spread of COVID-19 at passenger screening checkpoints, but its monitoring is not systematic or complete. Systematic and complete monitoring would improve TSA's assurance that its TSOs are appropriately implementing the procedural changes it has developed to reduce the spread of COVID-19. Moreover, we found that while TSA has some efforts underway to identify implementation trends, they are not leveraging available data to identify implementation trends across all airports. We identified additional sources of data (e.g., CCTV footage) that could be used to do such analysis, which would allow TSA to identify common concerns, challenges, and successes related to COVID-19 procedures at the nation's commercial airports. Using this information, TSA could also follow up to discover how field staff supported such successes, or respond to deficiencies with additional training, guidance, or other corrective intervention to help ensure correct nationwide implementation.

Recommendations for Executive Action

We are making the following two recommendations to TSA:

The TSA Administrator should take steps to ensure more complete monitoring of TSO implementation of measures to reduce the spread of infectious diseases at screening checkpoints. (Recommendation 1)

The TSA Administrator should take steps to analyze available data related to the implementation of its COVID-19 measures to identify patterns of successes and failures across all airports, and use its findings to share lessons learned and remediate any deficiencies. (Recommendation 2)

Agency Comments and Our Analysis

We provided a draft of this product to TSA for comment. In its comments, reproduced in appendix III, TSA concurred with our recommendations. TSA also provided technical comments, which we incorporated as appropriate.

With regard to our first recommendation that TSA take steps to ensure more complete monitoring of its measures to prevent the spread of infectious disease, TSA said its Enterprise Support Office and TSA's Security and Administrative Services, in coordination with the agency's Chief Medical Officer and Security Operations, will update TSA's COVID- 19 Standard Operating Procedures to require the implementation of the ICM position and associated data collection. Among other things, TSA said this effort will include updates to the ICM checklist to help verify that TSOs are complying with TSA's pandemic operating procedures, including correctly wearing personal protective equipment and social distancing between TSOs and passengers; an evaluation of data collection methods using the ICM checklist prior to system-wide implementation; and a quarterly assessment of the COVID-19 threat and whether TSA should continue or cease the ICM function. In addition, some of TSA's planned actions in response to this recommendation, such as considering whether to add the ICM position to its base plan, would enhance its preparation for future pandemics. TSA plans to complete these activities by the end of October 2021. If implemented effectively, these activities would address the intent of our recommendation.

With regard to our second recommendation that TSA take steps to analyze available data related to the implementation of COVID-19 measures to identify patterns of successes and failures across all airports, TSA said its Enterprise Support Office will work with the Security Operations, Performance Management Branch, to analyze available data, focusing on information captured from ICM checklists. TSA plans to complete these actions by the end of the December 2021, and will use results to identify areas for improvement and best practices to reduce the spread of infectious diseases at airport checkpoints. If implemented effectively, these activities would address the intent of our recommendation.

We are sending copies of this report to the appropriate congressional committees, the Secretary of Homeland Security and other interested parties.

In addition, the report is available at no charge on the GAO website at http://www.gao.gov.

If you or your staff have any questions about this report, please contact me at (202) 512-8777 or McNeilT@gao.gov. Contact points for our Office of Congressional Relations and Public Affairs may be found on the last page of this report. Key contributors to this report are listed in appendix IV.

Triana McNeil
Director, Homeland Security and Justice

List of Committees

The Honorable Patrick Leahy
Chairman
The Honorable Richard Shelby
Vice Chairman
Committee on Appropriations
United States Senate

The Honorable Ron Wyden
Chairman
The Honorable Mike Crapo
Ranking Member Committee on Finance
United States Senate

The Honorable Patty Murray
Chair
The Honorable Richard Burr
Ranking Member
Committee on Health, Education, Labor, and Pensions
United States Senate

The Honorable Gary C. Peters
Chair
The Honorable Rob Portman
Ranking Member
Committee on Homeland Security and Governmental Affairs
United States Senate

The Honorable Rosa L. DeLauro
Chairwoman
The Honorable Kay Granger
Ranking Member
Committee on Appropriations
House of Representatives
The Honorable Frank Pallone, Jr.
Chairman
The Honorable Cathy McMorris Rodgers
Republican Leader
Committee on Energy and Commerce
House of Representatives

The Honorable Bennie G. Thompson
Chairman
The Honorable John Katko
Ranking Member
Committee on Homeland Security
House of Representatives

The Honorable Carolyn B. Maloney
Chairwoman
The Honorable James Comer
Ranking Member
Committee on Oversight and Reform
House of Representatives

The Honorable Richard Neal
Chair
The Honorable Kevin Brady
Republican Leader, Committee on Ways and Means
House of Representatives

Appendix I: Objectives, Scope, and Methodology

The CARES Act—signed in March 2020—includes a provision for us to conduct monitoring and oversight of the federal government's efforts to prepare for, respond to, and recover from the COVID-19 pandemic.[1] In addition, we were asked to examine the Transportation Security Administration's (TSA) efforts to reduce human-to-human contact at airport passenger screening checkpoints in response to the Coronavirus Disease 2019 (COVID-19). This report assesses the following objectives:

1. How many Transportation Security Officers (TSO) have been diagnosed with COVID-19?
2. To what extent has TSA taken steps to reduce the spread of COVID-19 at passenger screening checkpoints?
3. How is TSA monitoring TSOs' implementation of the amended safety and screening procedures intended to reduce the spread of COVID-19 at passenger screening checkpoints?
4. How has TSA coordinated with other stakeholders to share and obtain information on steps taken to reduce the spread of COVID-19 at passenger screening checkpoints, and what have been the results?

Our review focused on those changes that were relevant to TSA's TSO employees, processes, and procedures in use at passenger screening checkpoints for roughly 440 commercial airports in the United States from January 2020 through January 2021.

In our background section, we analyzed publicly available TSA data on the number of passengers screened by TSA through checkpoints from March

[1] Pub. L. No. 116-136, § 19010, 134 Stat. 281, 579.

1, 2020 through January 31, 2021, as well as one calendar year prior. To assess the reliability of these data, we electronically reviewed the data for missing data and obvious errors. We found these data to be sufficiently reliable for the purposes of describing passenger throughput during the pandemic.

To address our first objective, we analyzed data received from TSA for the period March 1, 2020 through January 31, 2021 showing the number of reported positive COVID-19 cases among TSOs.[2] This data included information on the location (airport and region) where these employees worked, as well as the pay period in which they reported their diagnosis to TSA leadership. We used this data to calculate the rate of COVID-19 infections by pay period, that is, the number of newly reported COVID-19 cases divided by the total number of TSOs in that pay period. We also used this data to explore the distribution of COVID-19 cases across airports according to their 1) security risk categories and 2) geographical regions.[3] To assess the reliability of these data, we reviewed documentation from TSA's relevant program offices regarding the systems used to collect and store the data; questioned TSA officials from relevant program offices regarding the reliability of the data received; and electronically tested the data for missing data and obvious errors. We found these data to be sufficiently reliable for the purposes of describing the distribution of COVID-19 cases among TSOs at the nation's airports.

To address our second objective, we reviewed key TSA policies and procedures enacted to reduce the spread of COVID-19, including reviewing Department of Homeland Security (DHS) and TSA documentation of 1) procedural changes enacted and any new tools and technologies employed at passenger screening checkpoints to reduce the need for TSOs to come in contact with passengers and their belongings and increase TSOs' ability to physically distance themselves from passengers and coworkers; 2) guidance on the use of personal protective equipment, such as surgical masks and N95

---

[2] TSA does not provide testing to its employees. However, it requires local TSA (or contractor) management to report confirmed cases of COVID-19 in their workforce by entering incident information into the electronic WebEOC system. The system allows for two types of confirmation: 1) the employee has signs and symptoms clinically compatible as identified by a healthcare provider, but employee was not tested; or was tested and the result is pending; 2) the employee received a laboratory-confirmed positive result. The system does not require management to indicate what type of testing was performed to determine the diagnosis.

[3] TSA oversees security checkpoints at approximately 440 TSA-regulated airports nationwide. TSA classifies airports into one of five security risk categories (X, I, II, III, IV) based on various factors, such as the total number of takeoffs and landings annually, and other special security considerations. In general, category X airports have the highest number of passenger boardings and category IV airports have the fewest.

respirators, nitrile gloves, face shields, and acrylic barriers; and (3) human capital policies and flexibilities, such as the addition of leave categories, amended leave policies, and expanded telework opportunities.[4]

We evaluated the extent to which these policies, procedures, tools, and technologies were consistent with TSA's *Incident Management Framework: Chemical/Biological and Pandemic Base Plan (b*ase plan) and that TSA's actions noted incorporation of guidance from the Centers for Disease Control and Prevention and with guidance from the Occupational Safety and Health Administration that provide standards for cleaning and disinfecting the workplace and the need for PPE for different occupations based on the risk to the employee.[5] We did not assess the extent to which these changes influenced the security effectiveness of TSA's screening procedures.[6]

Also to address our second objective, we reviewed TSA time and attendance data to understand TSOs' use of expanded leave and telework flexibilities. To assess the reliability of these data, we reviewed documentation from TSA's relevant program offices regarding the systems used to collect and store the data; questioned TSA officials from relevant program offices regarding the reliability of the data received; and electronically tested the data for missing data and obvious errors. We found that the TSA time and attendance data was sufficiently reliable for the purpose of describing TSO's use of different leave and time charges during the time period under study.

In addition, to address our second objective, we conducted 21 interviews with aviation stakeholders about their experience with TSA's guidance and other tools to reduce the spread of COVID-19. These stakeholders included TSA Federal Security Directors (FSDs), airport operator officials, and TSO union representatives at a non-generalizable sample of commercial airports. We chose 8 of 440 commercial airports that 1) had variation in the number of confirmed cases of COVID-19 among TSOs or contract screeners; 2)

---

[4] Surgical masks are loosely fitting masks that help block large particle droplets and splatter from reaching the wearer's nose and mouth and that reduce the exposure of other's to the wearer's saliva and secretions. N95 respirators are tight fitting face pieces that requires a proper seal, which forces inhaled air to be pulled through the respirator's filter material. They are used to filter smaller airborne contaminants.

[5] For CDC guidance, See https://www.cdc.gov/coronavirus/2019-ncov/community/worker-safety-support/airports.html. For OSHA Guidance see *Guidance on Preparing Workplaces for COVID-19*, OSHA 3990-03 2020, and https://www.osha.gov/coronavirus/control-prevention/border-protection-transportation-sec urity, respectively.

[6] TSA assessed all proposed changes to TSA's standard operating procedures to ensure none would have a negative impact on security. As a result of its assessment, it did not implement two of the proposed changes because it determined they would pose a significant risk to security. These changes related to TSOs' handling of passenger identification and pat-downs.

represented diverse geographic areas; and 3) represented a variety of categories (an indicator of size).[7] In addition, one of our eight sample airports was a participant in TSA's Screening Partnership program.[8] We spoke to FSDs at all eight of our sample airports; officials from the airport operator at six, and union officials from five.[9]

Additionally, for our Screening Partnership Program airport, we chose to speak to officials from the private company that provides the airport's screening services about their experiences working with TSA leadership and how they implemented COVID-19 related changes at their checkpoints. In order to ensure we heard more than one private company perspective, we also spoke to the Screening Partnership Program company operating at the spoke of one of our sample airports. While results from these interviews are not representative, and therefore cannot be used to make inferences about a population, they do provide important context and illustrative examples. For example, interviews provided important insight from the viewpoints of field employees about 1) how TSA leadership communicated policy and procedural

---

[7] TSA's national operations are divided into seven geographic regions across the country. TSA has recently revised its field structure by reducing its geographic regions from seven to five. In the newstructure, TSA combined regions 2 and 7. It also divided region 5 states across other regions, moving Washington, Oregon, and Idaho to region 6, and Montana, Wyoming, Colorado, Utah, and the Dakotas to region 4. For the purposes of this report, we use the previous seven-region structure since that is how TSA provided data tous. FSDs represent a number of airports, including "hub" airports as well as their "spokes." Hubs are generally the larger category X or I airports, and many hubs have one or more spokes that are generally smaller category II, III, and IV airports. We chose some airports that had smaller spoke airports that had experienced cases of COVID-19. We wanted to ensure that we heard from FSDs about how smaller airports implemented procedural changes to reduce the spread of the disease. For example, one of our sample airports was Orlando International Airport (category X), and its FSD also discussed experiences from its spoke, Orlando Sanford (category II).

[8] Federal law established this program in 2001, originally as a pilot program and then on a permanent basis, to allow commercial airports to use TSA-approved qualified private-screening contractors to screen passengers and property. 49 U.S.C. § 44920. As of April 2021, contractors perform passenger and baggage screening services at 22 airports across the country. At each of these airports, TSA continues to be responsible for overseeing screening operations, and the contractors must adhere to TSA's security standards, procedures, and requirements.

[9] We originally selected a sample of six airports. Partway through the review, we selected an additional two airports that had not experienced any cases of COVID-19 among its TSOs to discover whether officials at these airports were taking markedly different approaches to the pandemic. We spoke to the FSDs at these airports because FSDs are the top ranking officials at airports implementing TSA policies to prevent COVID-19. Based on these interviews, we found that the two airports were not pursuing markedly different approaches to those we learned about; in addition, soon after we spoke to them, these two airports had their first cases among TSOs. Given that these airports were not substantially different than the others in our sample, we determined it was not necessary to interview airport operators or union officials.

changes, 2) the extent to which policies and procedural changes were being implemented successfully in the field, and 3) the challenges that field employees and airport operators faced as they implemented these changes.

To address our third objective, we reviewed TSA internal and published plans to assess the implementation of and compliance with procedures to reduce the spread of COVID-19 at airports' passenger screening checkpoints. For example, we reviewed the checklist provided to field employees for tracking the availability of personal protective equipment (PPE), the proper use of PPE, and TSO efforts to maintain physical distance from passengers, among other checklist items. We examined the extent to which this checklist was consistent with TSA's policies and procedural changes related to COVID-19. We also interviewed TSA headquarters officials about any challenges associated with monitoring the implementation and effectiveness of these procedures. As discussed above, we spoke with FSDs, airport operator officials, and union representatives from a non-generalizable sample of airports to understand any local airport efforts to monitor compliance and to obtain local officials' views on TSA headquarters' efforts to monitor compliance. We assessed the extent to which TSA's efforts to monitor the implementation of these procedural changes are consistent with its base plan and the Project Management Institute's *The Standard for Program Management.*[10] This guidance, which is used worldwide, describes principles, practices, and activities of program management that are generally recognized to support good program management practices and that are applicable to most programs, most of the time. In addition, the information and communication component of internal controls was significant to this objective, along with its related principle that management should use quality information to achieve its objectives.[11] We assessed the extent to which TSA's monitoring efforts reflected this principle.

Also to address our third objective, we observed CCTV footage from six selected airports to observe whether these airports were properly implementing the changes to policies and procedures that TSA instituted.[12] We requested files showing a variety of angles across the screening checkpoint: 1) the travel document checker area, including queueing areas; 2) divestment; 3) the walk-through metal detector and advanced imaging

---

[10] Project Management Institute, Inc., *The Standard for Program Management*, Fourth Edition.

[11] GAO, *Standards for Internal Control in the Federal Government*, GAO-14-704G (Washington, D.C.: Sept. 2014).

[12] We requested CCTV footage from the original six sample airports, which had more COVID-19 cases than the remaining two airports we spoke with.

technology machines, including angles showing pat- downs and use of explosives trace detection machines for on-person searches; 4) recomposure; and 5) the carry-on bag search area and use of explosives trace detection machines for in-property searches. We requested CCTV footage at two different time periods—the first set was captured between July and August 2020 and the second in December 2020—in order to observe whether there were meaningful changes in compliance over the course of the pandemic. We received more than 100 hours of footage from our sample airports. We selected and reviewed the first ten minutes of footage showing each of the above-listed angles from each airport.[13] For each file, one analyst reviewed the footage and captured the timestamps and details for one or more examples of TSA's required and recommended procedural changes being implemented properly and improperly on an Excel spreadsheet. The changes the analyst looked for are summarized in Table 1.

Table 1. Examples of Transportation Security Administration (TSA) Requirements and Recommended Practices to Reduce the Spread of COVID-19 at Checkpoints that GAO Examined in Closed-Circuit Television (CCTV) Footage from Six Sample Airports

Reduced Touch Points	The credential authentication technology machine is rotated for passenger self-service
	TSOs allow passengers who alarm to further divest and rescreen
Presence of Signage and Use of Barriers	Floor decals emphasizing physical distancing recommendations throughout the checkpoint
	Other signage visible related to COVID-19 precautions
	Plexiglass installed to protect TSOs and passengers throughout the checkpoint
Evidence of Physical Distance Being Maintained	Between passengers and TSOs throughout the checkpoint
	Among TSOs throughout the checkpoint
TSO Use of Personal Protective Equipment	Surgical masks
	Face shields
	Nitrile gloves
	Changing gloves following on-person searches
	Discarding explosives trace detection swabs after a single use

Source: GAO analysis. | GAO-21-364.

Notes: We reviewed CCTV footage from six sample airports.

[13] We did not request footage from specific days or times but believe the footage we selected and reviewed was sufficiently reliable for our purposes of observing whether airports were properly implementing the changes to policies and procedures TSA implemented during the pandemic.

Once the analyst reviewed the footage and captured relevant timestamps, a second analyst reviewed the footage and indicated whether they agreed with the first analyst's assessment (i.e., implemented properly vs implemented improperly). If they did not initially agree, they discussed the timestamp and came to an agreement. Although results from the review of this footage from selected airports are not representative, and therefore cannot be used to make inferences about a population, they do provide important context and illustrative examples. For example, reviewing this footage allowed us to observe 1) examples of how TSOs in the field were implementing COVID-19 procedural changes; 2) examples of inconsistent implementation across our sample airports; and 3) the utility of CCTV footage as a monitoring tool that TSA leadership could leverage.

To address our fourth objective, we reviewed TSA documentation of its efforts to share and obtain information with industry, federal, and domestic and international airport stakeholders on any new policies, procedures, tools, and technologies to reduce the spread of COVID-19 that could be employed at U.S. airports' passenger screening checkpoints. Specifically, we reviewed TSA documentation summarizing its COVID-related international interagency coordination as well as multiple TSA press releases outlining steps the agency is taking to help mitigate the impact of COVID-19 on travelers and its workforce. To understand how TSA is working with federal partners to share and obtain information on technologies and tools to reduce the spread of COVID-19, we interviewed officials from TSA's Requirements and Capabilities Analysis office and DHS's Science and Technology Directorate (S&T).[14] To understand how TSA is working with aviation industry stakeholders, we interviewed officials from the industry groups Airlines for America and the Airports Council International to discuss how they have communicated with TSA to share information about technologies or procedures that their membership is using or planning to use to reduce the spread of COVID-19.[15] We selected these industry groups because they are members of TSAs Aviation Security Advisory Committee and represent the

[14] TSA's Requirements and Capabilities Analysis office directly supports TSA's mission by assessing current state operations, conducting gap analyses, managing needs identification, and developing requirements to generate new and improved security capabilities in alignment with the future vision of aviation security.

[15] Airlines for America is a trade association that works with member airlines, labor, Congress, and other groups to improve the aviation industry. Airports Council International advocates for policies and provides services for more than 300 local, regional, and state commercial airport owners and operators in the United States and Canada.

leading passenger and cargo carriers in the U.S. and more than 300 airport owners and operators, respectively.

To understand how TSA is working with domestic airport stakeholders, we interviewed FSDs, officials from airport operators, and union officials at the non-generalizable sample of domestic airports described above. Finally, to understand how TSA is working with foreign airport stakeholders, we interviewed Transportation Security Administration Representatives posted at a judgmentally selected sample of four international regions.[16] We selected these regions to obtain geographic diversity among the airports with TSA Representatives. Although results from these interviews cannot be generalized to all TSA Representatives who serve internationally, they do provide important context and illustrative examples. For example, interviews with officials knowledgeable about operations at domestic and international airports provided insight on TSA efforts to learn about promising practices, technologies, or tools employed in the U.S. and abroad. Finally, to determine the extent to which TSA has participated in the development of key international aviation sector guidance, we interviewed officials from the International Civil Aviation Organization.

We conducted this performance audit from May 2020 to June 2021 in accordance with generally accepted government auditing standards. Those standards require that we plan and perform the audit to obtain sufficient, appropriate evidence to provide a reasonable basis for our findings and conclusions based on our audit objectives. We believe that the evidence obtained provides a reasonable basis for our findings and conclusions based on our audit objectives.

Appendix II: Transportation Security Administration (TSA) Actions in Response to the Coronavirus Disease 2019 Pandemic

TSA took steps to address the spread of COVID-19 among its Transportation Security Officers (TSO) and travelers at checkpoints through staff communication, management actions, and procedural and human capital

---

[16] Transportation Security Administration Representatives are TSA officials who are posted at US embassies and consulates abroad. They serve as TSA's interlocutors to foreign governments and advisors to Ambassadors and Chiefs of Mission on aviation security issues. They engage with counterparts, including foreign airports, and facilitate information exchange and dialogue.

changes. The following figures show TSA's key actions in each of these areas relative to pandemic milestones.

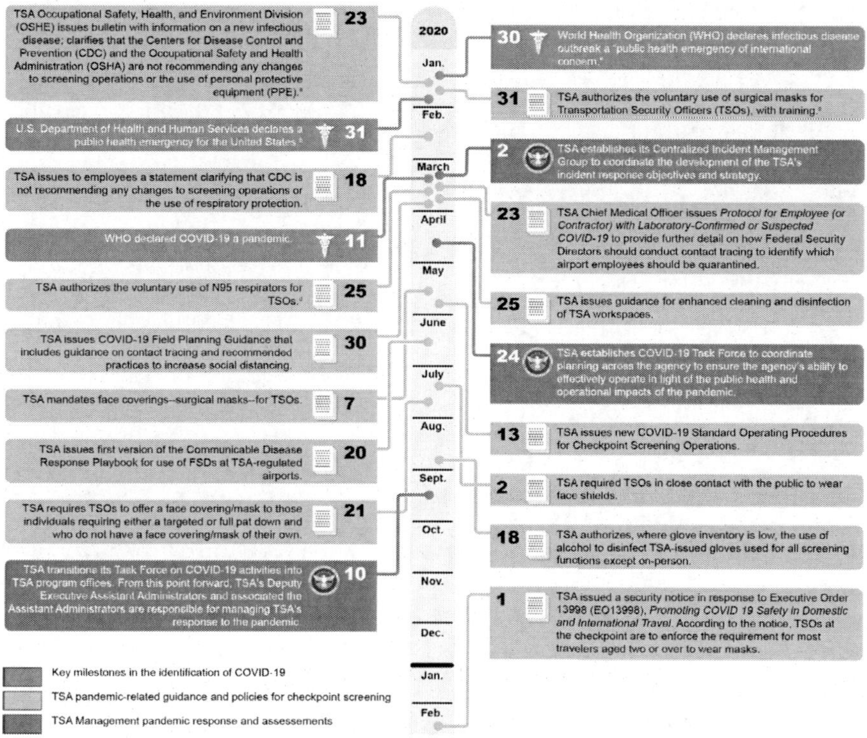

Source: GAO analysis of TSA information. | GAO-21-364.

[a]PPE include masks, gloves, face shields and other equipment workers use to protect themselves from the transmission of infectious diseases that could occur during the performance of activities.

[b]A public health of emergency is declared to respond to a significant outbreak of an infectious disease, bioterrorist attack, or other significant or catastrophic event.

[c]Surgical masks are loosely fitting masks that help block large particle droplets and splatter from reaching the wearer's nose and mouth and that reduce the exposure of others to the wearer's saliva and secretions.

[d]N95 respirators are tight fitting face pieces that require a proper seal, which forces inhaled air to be pulled through the respirator's filter material. They are used to filter smaller airborne contaminants.

Figure 15. Coronavirus Disease 2019 (COVID-19) Pandemic Milestones and Key Transportation Security Administration (TSA) Management Actions and Guidance Changes, January 2020 to February 2021.

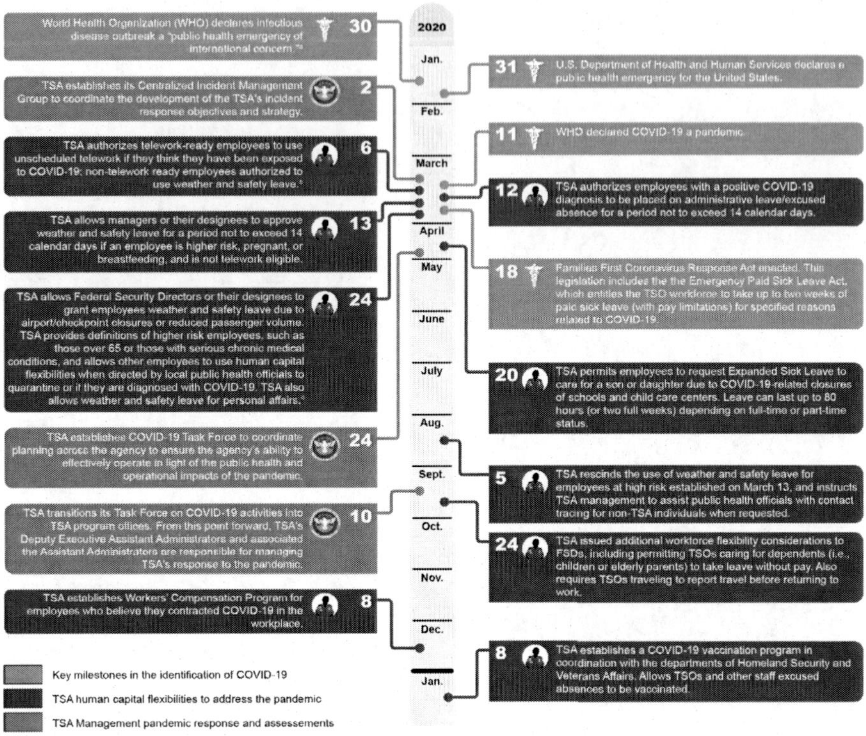

Source: GAO analysis of TSA information. | GAO-21-364.

[a]A public health of emergency is declared to respond to a significant outbreak of an infectious disease, bioterrorist attack, or other significant or catastrophic.

[b]TSA allows for the approval of weather and safety leave, a form of paid leave, if an employee (or a group of employees) is prevented from safely traveling to or performing work at an approved location.

[c]Federal Security Directors (FSD) are responsible for ensuring TSA policies and procedures are carried out locally at airports.

Figure 16. Coronavirus Disease 2019 (COVID-19) Pandemic Milestones and Key Transportation Security Administration (TSA) Management Actions and Human Capital Policy Changes, January 2020 to January 2021.

Appendix III: Comments from the Department of Homeland Security

U.S. Department of Homeland Security
Washington, DC 20528

Homeland Security

May 27, 2021

Triana McNeil
Director, Homeland Security and Justice
U.S. Government Accountability Office
441 G Street, NW
Washington, DC 20548

Re: Management Response to Draft Report: GAO-21-364, "COVID-19: TSA Could Better Monitor Its Efforts to Reduce Infectious Disease Spread at Checkpoints"

Dear Ms. McNeil:

Thank you for the opportunity to comment on this draft report. The U.S. Department of Homeland Security (DHS or the Department) appreciates the U.S. Government Accountability Office's (GAO) work in planning and conducting its review and issuing this report.

The Department is pleased to note GAO's positive recognition that in January 2020, when the U.S. experienced its first cases of the COVID-19 virus, the Transportation Security Administration (TSA) began coordinating its response to the pandemic and implementing an array of changes to reduce the spread of COVID-19 at airport checkpoints. This included issuing amended safety measures, such as requiring Transportation Security Officers (TSOs) to wear surgical masks and face shields, change gloves after pat-downs, and physically distance themselves from coworkers and passengers, as practicable. TSA also appreciates GAO's feedback that TSOs, union officials, and other stakeholders were generally satisfied with TSA's efforts. TSA remains committed to reducing the spread of COVID-19 at airport passenger screening checkpoints by continuing to implement safety measures, as appropriate, in partnership with its aviation stakeholders.

The draft report contained two recommendations, with which the Department concurs. Attached find our detailed response to each recommendation. DHS previously submitted technical comments addressing several accuracy, contextual, sensitivity, and other issues under a separate cover for GAO's consideration.

Again, thank you for the opportunity to review and comment on this draft report. Please feel free to contact me if you have any questions. We look forward to working with you again in the future.

Sincerely,

JIM H CRUMPACKER Digitally signed by JIM H CRUMPACKER Date: 2021.05.27 16:34:02 -04'00'

JIM H. CRUMPACKER, CIA, CFE
Director
Departmental GAO-OIG Liaison Office

Attachment

Attachment: Management Response to Recommendations Contained in GAO-21-364; 104290

GAO recommended that the TSA Administrator:

Recommendation 1: Take steps to ensure more complete monitoring of TSO implementation of measures to reduce the spread of infectious diseases at screening checkpoints.

Response: Concur. Although the Infection Control Monitor (ICM) position was previously established in June 2020 as a best management practice, TSA's Enterprise Support Office and TSA's Security and Administrative Services (SAS), in coordination with the agency's Chief Medical Officer and Security Operations, will also update TSA's COVID-19 Standard Operating Procedures that require the implementation of the ICM and associated data collection. Once complete, this update will deliver:

- A recommendation to the TSA Administrator as to whether TSA should require ICM implementation as part of a broader pandemic preparedness policy including criteria for implementing and implementing guidelines.
- Adding the ICM position to TSA's "Incident Management Framework: Chemical/Biological and Pandemic Base Plan" as part of TSA's response and recovery efforts during future pandemics.
- Updates to the ICM checklist which will increase TSA's ability to verify that personnel comply with TSA's pandemic operating procedures, including correctly wearing Personal Protective Equipment and social distancing between TSOs and passengers.
- An evaluation of the: (1) method of data collection; (2) system that is used to collect it; (3) frequency of ICM checklist use; and (4) a recommendation to the TSA Administrator as to the implementation and use of the ICM checklist, including a plan for piloting its use prior to system-wide implementation.
- A quarterly assessment of the evolving COVID-19 threat, as well as a recommendation as to whether TSA should continue or cease use of the ICM checklist procedure, in accordance with any updates to the ICM policy and the "Incident Management Framework: Chemical/Biological and Pandemic Base Plan."

Estimated Completion Date (ECD): October 29, 2021.

Recommendation 2: Take steps to analyze available data related to the implementation of its COVID-19 measures to identify patterns of successes and failures across all airports and use its findings to share lessons learned and remediate any deficiencies.

Response: Concur. TSA's Enterprise Support Office will work with the Security Operations, Performance Management Branch, to analyze available data to identify patterns of success and failure in implementing COVID-19 measures across airports nationwide. In addition, TSA's SAS will provide training and guidance to Security Operations by engaging Designated Occupational Safety and Health Officials based on ICM data related to their COVID-19 implementation measures. SAS will use this data to improve processes to reduce the spread of infectious diseases at checkpoints, focusing on using existing data captured on the ICM checklist to identify weaknesses and outstanding performers, and sharing best practices to increase the overall effectiveness.

ECD: December 31, 2021.

Appendix IV: Staff Acknowledgments

In addition to the contact named above, Mona Nichols Blake (Assistant Director), Anthony DeFrank (Analyst in Charge), Landis Lindsey, Sarah Williamson, Mariel Alper, Paul Aussendorf, Benjamin Crossley, Elizabeth Dretsch, David Hooper, Sara Ann Moessbauer, Moon Parks, Jasmine Porter, and Adam Vogt made key contributions to this report.

Chapter 3

COVID-19: Federal Air Marshal Service Should Document Its Response to Cases and Facilitate Access to Testing*

United States Government Accountability Office

Abbreviations

CDC	Centers for Disease Control and Prevention
COVID-19	Coronavirus Disease 2019
DHS	Department of Homeland Security
FAMS	Federal Air Marshal Service
PPE	Personal Protective Equipment
SAC	Supervisory Air Marshal in Charge
TSA	Transportation Security Administration
VIPR	Visible Intermodal Prevention and Response

Why GAO Did This Study

In the U.S. there have been over 29 million cumulative reported cases of COVID-19 and about 524,000 reported deaths, as of March 23, 2021. Public health officials have recommended social distancing and other steps to reduce the spread of the disease, but air marshals often work on planes where they cannot fully adopt these measures. The CARES Act included a provision for GAO to conduct monitoring and oversight of the federal government's response to the COVID- 19 pandemic. This report examines (1) how many air marshals have been diagnosed with COVID-19; (2) FAMS's steps to protect

* This is an edited, reformatted and augmented version of the United States Government Accountability Office Report to Congressional Committees, Publication No. GAO-21-595, dated June 2021.

air marshals' health; and (3) how FAMS adapted its operations during the pandemic.

GAO analyzed FAMS data on COVID- 19 cases among employees, reviewed agency guidance, analyzed FAMS flight operations reports, and interviewed FAMS leadership as well as air marshals at a non-generalizable sample of three field offices selected for variation in number of COVID-19 cases, among other things. This is a public version of a sensitive report that GAO issued in May 2021. Information that DHS deemed sensitive has been omitted.

What GAO Recommends

GAO recommends that FAMS (1) consistently document steps taken in response to an employee's diagnosis with COVID-19 and (2) routinely facilitate employee access to testing for COVID-19. DHS concurred with both of GAO's recommendations and identified actions it will take to implement them.

What GAO Found

The U.S. Federal Air Marshal Service (FAMS), within the Department of Homeland Security (DHS), reported 345 cases of COVID-19 among employees, as of January 31, 2021.

To protect air marshals from COVID-19, FAMS provided supplies like N95 masks and implemented new telework and leave policies. FAMS also created protocols for responding to employees with COVID-19, but has not consistently documented their implementation. By doing so, FAMS could better ensure it is taking the required steps to protect employees and the flying public. GAO also found FAMS does not routinely facilitate employee access to COVID-19 testing. FAMS recommends employees seek testing through their medical provider or local public health officials, but air marshals in all three field offices GAO met with either noted barriers to testing or benefits to improved access to tests. In January 2021, FAMS employees became eligible for COVID-19 vaccinations, but Centers for Disease Control and Prevention guidance says testing continues to be important even as vaccinations become available. By facilitating access to testing, FAMS could better ensure employee health and continued operations.

Federal Air Marshal Service's Reported Cases of COVID-19, as of January 31, 2021

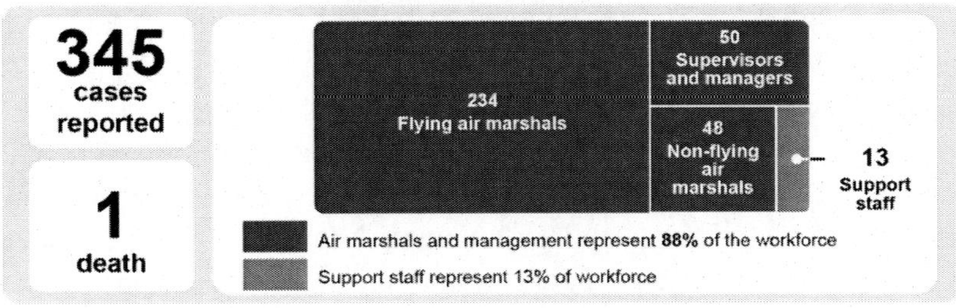

Source: GAO analysis of Federal Air Marshal Service data. | GAO-21-595.
Note: Cases included in the figure were confirmed with a positive COVID-19 test and reported to the Federal Air Marshal Service by the employee.

Starting in February 2020, FAMS adjusted the number and types of flights air marshals covered. In April 2020, amidst a decline in U.S. carrier flights, the number of flights FAMS covered declined by 90 percent compared to average monthly flights pre-pandemic. By June 2020, FAMS had resumed pre-pandemic flight levels. From April through August 2020, FAMS made operational changes to increase its flight coverage that also resulted in FAMS covering different types of flights, compared to those it covered prior to the pandemic. For example, due to travel restrictions, FAMS stopped covering most international flights but increased coverage of other types of flights. Starting in April 2020, FAMS also increased air marshals' non-flight work, such as providing a security presence at airports and national events.

June 23, 2021
Congressional Committees

The Coronavirus Disease 2019 (COVID-19) has resulted in catastrophic loss of life. In the U.S., as of March 23, 2021, there were about 29.7 million cumulative reported cases and more than 524,000 reported deaths, according to federal agencies.[1] Public health officials have recommended social

[1] Data on COVID-19 cases in the U.S. are based on aggregate case reporting to the Centers for Disease Control and Prevention (CDC) and include probable and confirmed cases as reported by states and jurisdictions. CDC's National Center for Health Statistics COVID-19 death counts in the U.S. are based on provisional counts from death certificate data, which do not distinguish between laboratory-confirmed and probable COVID-19 deaths.

distancing and other measures to reduce transmission of the disease. However, certain sectors of the U.S. workforce with critical roles such as in law enforcement and transportation have remained at risk of catching and spreading the virus because their jobs require that they come into regular contact with other people. The U.S. Federal Air Marshal Service (FAMS)—an office within the Department of Homeland Security's (DHS) Transportation Security Administration (TSA)—is one such workforce.[2]

FAMS is tasked with promoting confidence in the nation's civil aviation system through the deployment of air marshals to protect U.S. air carriers, airports, passengers, and crews. To accomplish this mission, FAMS deploys armed federal law enforcement officers—air marshals—to provide an onboard security presence on selected flights of U.S. air carriers travelling within the U.S. and around the world.[3] FAMS's mission has continued throughout the COVID-19 pandemic with air marshals routinely working on airplanes and at airports; flying domestic and international routes. The Department of State has advised U.S. citizens to avoid international travel and the Centers for Disease Control and Prevention (CDC) has warned that with regard to COVID-19, high-risk settings include workplaces where physical distancing is difficult and workers are in close contact with coworkers or the public.[4] As such, COVID-19 presents a particular health concern for flying air marshals and the public with whom they interact in the course of their work.

The CARES Act—signed in March 2020—includes a provision for us to conduct monitoring and oversight of the federal government's efforts to prepare for, respond to, and recover from the COVID-19 pandemic.[5] In addition, we were asked to review the steps DHS is taking to protect its employees from contracting COVID-19, among other things. This report examines, (1) how many air marshals have been diagnosed with COVID- 19;

Provisional counts are incomplete due to an average delay of 2 weeks (a range of 1–8 weeks or longer) for death certificate processing. The data were accessed on March 23, 2021. Data include deaths occurring from January 2020 through the week ending on March 20, 2021.

[2] The formal name of this office is Law Enforcement / Federal Air Marshal Service, but we refer to it as the Federal Air Marshal Service throughout this report.

[3] See 49 U.S.C. § 44917.

[4] CDC "SARS-CoV-2 Testing Strategy: Considerations for Non-Healthcare Workplaces, Testing in Non-Healthcare Workplaces." July 22, 2020. Accessed October 14, 2020, https://www.cdc.gov/coronavirus/2019-ncov/community/organizations/testing-non-healthcare-workplaces.html.

[5] Pub. L. No. 116-136, § 19010, 134 Stat. 281, 579. We regularly issue government-wide reports on the federal response to COVID-19. For the latest report, see GAO, *COVID-19: Sustained Federal Action Is Crucial as Pandemic Enters Its Second Year,* GAO-21-387 (Washington, D.C.: Mar. 31, 2021). Our next government-wide report will be issued in July 2021 and will be available on GAO's website at https://www.gao.gov/coronavirus.

(2) FAMS's steps to protect air marshals' health during the COVID-19 pandemic; and (3) how FAMS has adapted its operations during the COVID-19 pandemic.

This report is a public version of the prior sensitive report that we issued in May 2021.[6] TSA deemed some of the information in our May report to be sensitive security information, which must be protected from public disclosure. Therefore, this report omits this information, such as the number of air marshals as well as data and details associated with FAMS's flight operations. Although the information provided in this report is more limited in scope, it addresses the same objectives as the sensitive report and uses the same methodology.

To address our first objective, we analyzed FAMS data and reports to identify the number of cases of COVID-19 among employees, as reported to FAMS management through January 31, 2021.[7] Specifically, we analyzed data collected by the FAMS Medical Programs Section—the office within FAMS tasked with monitoring cases of COVID-19—to track reported cases of COVID-19 among the workforce.[8] We also analyzed periodic reports summarizing new cases for FAMS management, as well as FAMS summary data on the number of cases broken out by employee location and employee type (i.e., flying air marshals, ground-based air marshals, etc.).[9] We assessed the reliability of these summary data by cross-checking totals from each source, matching totals for the breakouts by field office location and employee type, and resolving discrepancies with FAMS officials. We also spoke with officials from FAMS management and FAMS's Medical Programs Section to

[6] GAO, *COVID-19: Federal Air Marshal Service Should Document Its Response to Cases and Facilitate Access to Testing*, GAO-21-382SU (Washington, D.C.: May 5, 2021).

[7] FAMS does not have information on whether employees caught COVID-19 through their work. The Department of Labor's Office of Workers' Compensation Programs has determined that for the purposes of the Federal Employees' Compensation Act, federal law enforcement officers—such as air marshals—whose employment causes them to come into direct and frequent in-person and close proximity contact with the public are assumed to have contracted COVID-19 as a result of their employment.

[8] In addition to tracking reported cases, the FAMS Medical Programs Section tracked employees' reported history of symptoms, the date the employee contacted the Section, the employee's field office location, whether the employee had a COVID-19 test, and the results of the test where known, among other things. This spreadsheet included over 700 employee symptom history records beginning February 16, 2020 through January 31, 2021. FAMS summarized employee reports of COVID-19 symptoms and cases in more than 50 reports for FAMS management, on a daily or weekly basis, beginning March 11, 2020 through January 31, 2021.

[9] In addition to conducting flight operations, air marshals may carry out the FAMS mission by participating in ground-based operational assignments that support security activities in transportation settings.

understand how they tracked and reported these data. We determined that these data were sufficiently reliable for describing the number of reported cases of COVID-19 among FAMS employees, including the employees' office locations and roles.[10]

To address our second objective, we reviewed TSA and FAMS COVID-19-specific guidance to identify changes in policy and procedure intended to protect employees from COVID-19, such as new procedures for contact tracing, among other steps. Specifically, we reviewed TSA's *Human Capital Advisory Memos (versions 1 through 8)*; TSA's August 2020 *Guidance for COVID-19: Return to Workplace and Medical Documentation*; and FAMS's July 2020 *COVID-19 Protocol for Assistant Administrators, Supervisory Air Marshal In Charge*, or *Federal Security Director (FAMS Protocols)*.[11] We also reviewed FAMS's, TSA's, and DHS's internal communications to employees during the period January 22, 2020 to August 6, 2020 related to COVID-19, such as email messages with best practices to avoid contracting COVID-19 during travel. Lastly, we compared the steps FAMS had taken to protect employees to CDC and Federal Occupational Safety and Health Administration guidance for workplaces responding to COVID-19 and considerations for COVID-19 testing in non-medical workplaces.[12]

To obtain FAMS officials' perspectives on the steps taken to protect employees from COVID-19 and how FAMS management is monitoring

---

[10] Throughout this report, the numbers of cases of COVID-19 among FAMS employees refers to confirmed cases where an employee received a COVID-19 test and reported their positive test result to the FAMS Medical Programs Section.

[11] TSA, Human Capital Advisory Memo 2020.30.4 (rev. 8); Appendix A – Return to Workplace and Medical Documentation; and Appendix B – Assistant Administrator (AA)/Supervisory Air Marshal in Charge (SAC)/ Federal Security Director (FSD) Protocol for Employee (or Contractor) with Laboratory-Confirmed or Suspected COVID-19.
December 8, 2020. According to FAMS management officials, the FAMS Protocols have been revised three times, since the first version issued on April 2, 2020. The Return to Workplace Documentation guidance was first issued July 2020. TSA has revised the Human Capital Advisory Memo eight times, to reflect changes in policies. Beginning with the seventh version (dated September 24, 2020), the Return to Workplace guidance and FAMS Protocols appear as appendix A and B respectively.

[12] CDC "Domestic Travel during the COVID-19 Pandemic." December 2, 2020. Accessed December 14, 2020, https://www.cdc.gov/coronavirus/2019-ncov/travelers/travel-during-covid19.html; CDC "Testing Strategy for Coronavirus (COVID-19) in High-Density Critical Infrastructure Workplaces after a COVID-19 Case is Identified, Testing in High-Density Critical Infrastructure Workplaces" June 13, 2020. Accessed October 14, 2020, https://www.cdc.gov/coronavirus/2019-ncov/community/worker-safety-support/hd-testing.html; Occupational Safety and Health Administration "Guidance on Preparing Workplaces for COVID-19." March 9, 2020, and Occupational Safety and Health Administration. "Protecting Workers: Guidance on Mitigating and Preventing the Spread of COVID-19 in the Workplace". January 29, 2021.

implementation of these steps, we interviewed senior FAMS management officials, including the Assistant Administrator for Field Operations and the Assistant Administrator for Flight Operations. We also interviewed field office management officials and air marshals in three of the 20 FAMS field office locations—Newark, New Jersey; Houston, Texas; and Seattle, Washington. We selected these field offices to capture perspectives from field offices that had experienced varying numbers of COVID-19 cases, as well as varied effects on their operations, such as decreased international flights.

We developed standardized lists of questions that we used in each of the three field offices to facilitate two separate discussion sessions—one with field office management officials, including the field office Supervisory Air Marshals in Charge (SAC), and the other with approximately five air marshals in each office. For the group discussion sessions with air marshals, we requested that each field office make available approximately five air marshals including both flying and non-flying air marshals. Although the information obtained from interviews with these officials is not generalizable to all 20 FAMS field offices, it provided insight into the steps FAMS had taken to protect air marshals' health during the pandemic and how these steps varied across offices.

We also met with representatives from the three external employee groups representing air marshals—the Air Marshal Association, the Air Marshal National Council, and the Federal Law Enforcement Officer Association—to obtain their perspectives on the steps FAMS had taken to protect air marshals from COVID-19 and whether additional steps were needed. We determined that the control activities component of internal control was significant to this objective, along with the underlying principle that management should design control activities to achieve objectives and respond to risks.[13] We assessed how FAMS has designed control activities to ensure implementation of the FAMS Protocols. We also compared FAMS's documentation requirements to *DHS Risk Management Fundamentals*—the purpose of which is to establish organizational practices that DHS components should follow to incorporate risk management into organizational missions.[14]

To address our third objective, we analyzed FAMS monthly flight operations reports from October 2019 through January 2021 to identify how FAMS's flight coverage—that is the number and types of flights FAMS

---

[13] GAO, *Standards for Internal Control in the Federal Government*, GAO-14-704G (Washington, D.C.: Sept. 2014).

[14] DHS, Risk Management Fundamentals: Homeland Security Risk Management Doctrine, (Washington, D.C.: April 2011).

covered—changed in response to the COVID-19 pandemic.[15] We assessed the reliability of the data presented in these reports by reviewing documentation and interviewing knowledgeable FAMS officials about their Aircrews and WebEOC flight tracking systems and how they ensure the quality of their data. We also compared FAMS's monthly flight operations reports to record-level flight data for the months of October 2019, April 2020, and January 2021 and resolved discrepancies through discussion with FAMS officials.[16] We determined that these data were sufficiently reliable for describing month-to-month changes in FAMS operations during this period. We also reviewed FAMS documentation of operational changes in response to COVID-19 and interviewed FAMS leadership about their decisions to make these changes. Further, we analyzed FAMS documentation of air marshals' ground-based (non-flight) activities from April 2020 through January 2021 and interviewed the Executive Assistant Administrator/Director of FAMS, the leadership, and three field office SACs about how FAMS's ground-based activities changed in response to the COVID-19 pandemic.

The performance audit upon which this report is based was conducted from July 2020 to May 2021 in accordance with generally accepted government auditing standards. Those standards require that we plan and perform the audit to obtain sufficient, appropriate evidence to provide a reasonable basis for our findings and conclusions based on our audit objectives. We believe that the evidence obtained provides a reasonable basis for our findings and conclusions based on our audit objectives. We subsequently worked with TSA from May through June 2021 to prepare this unclassified version of the original sensitive report for public release. This public version was also prepared in accordance with these standards.

Background

[15] To enable us to compare FAMS flight operations pre- and post-pandemic, we analyzed data for the period October 2019—the beginning of fiscal year 2020—through January 2021—the most recent month for which data were available at the time of our review.
Throughout our report, we use the term pre-pandemic to refer to flight data we reviewed for the period October 2019 through February 2020.

[16] Aircrews is FAMS's primary system for tracking flights and air marshal deployments. However, FAMS also captures some types of flights—namely top priority flights—in a second data system called WebEOC. In both systems, record-level flight data included details such as the flight departure and destination locations, the flight's FAMS-designated priority level, and whether or not air marshals covered the flight, among others.

FAMS Management

The senior leader of FAMS is the Executive Assistant Administrator/ Director of FAMS. FAMS management is organized into three divisions:

- Field Operations Division. Led by the Assistant Administrator for Field Operations, this division manages FAMS's 20 field offices located near major airports across the U.S. Each field office is managed by a SAC, assisted by a Deputy Supervisory Air Marshal in Charge or Assistant Supervisory Air Marshal in Charge, depending onthe size of the field office. The SACs are responsible for the day-to- day management of air marshals assigned to their field office.
- Flight Operation Division. Led by the Assistant Administrator for Flight Operations, this division is responsible for planning and preparing air marshals' schedules, monitoring all FAMS flights, and providing support to air marshals during flight operations.
- Operations Management Division. Led by the Assistant Administrator for Operations Management, this division is responsible for the agency-wide human capital and financial management of FAMS. Within this division, a staff of one part-time doctor and three occupational health nurses comprise the FAMS Medical Programs Section, located at FAMS's facility in Atlantic City, New Jersey.17 This unit is responsible for determining air marshals' medical fitness for duty, based on the results of required annual physicals completed by the air marshals' personal physicians. The doctor and nurses also respond to medical questions from air marshals, including questions about new health threats such as COVID-19, among other things.

FAMS Workforce

As of January 2021, FAMS had thousands of employees, the majority of whom are air marshals who conduct flight operations and other law enforcement work. The remainder of the FAMS workforce consists of administrative and mission support staff across their headquarters, field office locations, and training facilities. In addition to conducting flight operations,

[17] The Medical Programs Section also includes three administrative staff and two occupational health nurse positions that are vacant as of January 2021.

air marshals may carry out the FAMS mission by participating in ground-based operational assignments that support security activities in transportation settings. For example, FAMS assigns air marshals to Visible Intermodal Prevention and Response (VIPR) teams in all of its 20 field offices. See figure 1 for the locations of FAMS's 20 field offices.

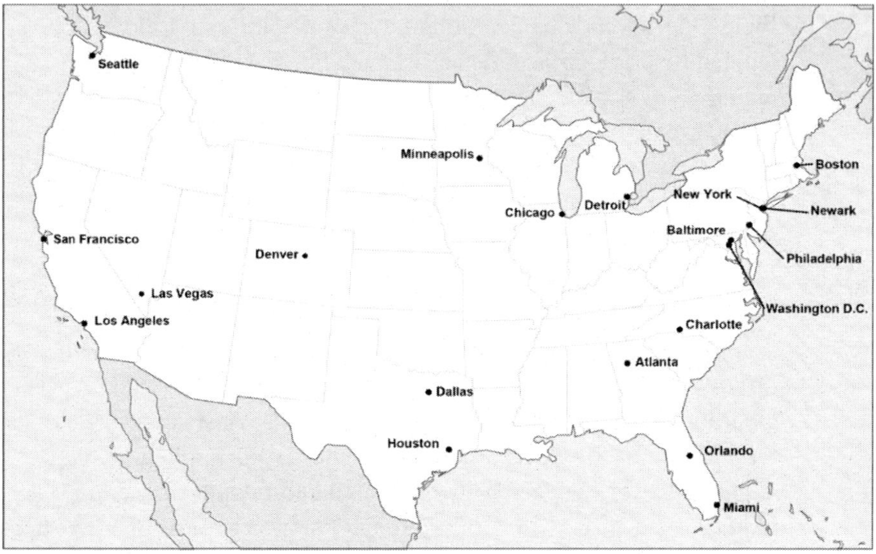

Source: GAO aummary of FAMSorganization. | GAO-21-595.

Note: This figure shows the locations of FAMS field offices. FAMS also has employees at its headquarters in Springfield, Virginia.

Figure 1. Location of Federal Air Marshal Service (FAMS) Field Offices.

VIPR teams consist of air marshals and other TSA security officers specializing in aviation, surface, and explosives inspections. VIPR teams deploy to provide a visible law enforcement and security screening presence at surface and maritime transportation locations, like public transit stations. In addition to VIPR teams, air marshals may support law enforcement operations at airports, such as conducting risk assessments of security threats. FAMS also deploys air marshals to provide support to other DHS components for a few days or several months, including the Federal Emergency Management Agency, U.S. Immigration and Customs Enforcement's Homeland Security Investigations, and the Secret Service.

In February 2020, we reported that the FAMS workforce had concerns about their health but FAMS had not comprehensively assessed the health of its workforce. We recommended that FAMS develop and implement a plan to assess the health and fitness of the FAMS workforce as a whole, including trends over time. DHS agreed with this recommendation and in January 2020, DHS officials stated that FAMS had established a team to develop a plan to do so, but as of January 2021, they had not taken further steps to implement the recommendation.[18]

FAMS's Concept of Operations

The Aviation and Transportation Security Act, enacted in November 2001, authorizes TSA to deploy air marshals on every passenger flight of a U.S. air carrier and requires TSA to deploy air marshals on every such flight determined by the TSA Administrator to present high security risks.[19] FAMS uses a concept of operations to set forth its methodology for deploying air marshals on flights.[20] FAMS prioritizes several categories of flights considered higher risk, including those for which a known or suspected terrorist is ticketed, called special mission coverage. FAMS further prioritizes deployment of air marshals on random, unpredictable flights, and supporting flights used to position air marshals for flights. (See table 1).[21]

Table 1. Categories of Flights the Federal Air Marshal Service (FAMS) Prioritizes

Category description	*Flight selection rationale*
Domestic: Certain flights within the U.S.	As resources permit, FAMS deploys air marshals on selected domestic flights.

[18] GAO, *Aviation Security: Federal Air Marshal Service Has Taken Steps to Address Workforce Issues, but Additional Actions Needed*, GAO-20-125 (Washington, D.C: Feb. 12, 2020). In addition to recommending that FAMS develop and implement a plan to assess the health and fitness of the FAMS workforce, we made five other recommendations to improve FAMS's tracking of employees' medical status, and strengthen efforts to prevent discrimination, among other things. DHS concurred with these recommendations, and as of January 2021, DHS had taken steps to address two of the six recommendations and had plans to implement the remaining four.

[19] See Pub. L. No. 107-71, § 105(a), 115 Stat. 597, 606; 49 U.S.C. § 44917(a)(1) and (2).

[20] FAMS may deploy air marshals on U.S. air carriers either operating within the U.S. or operating internationally if an agreement is in place with a destination country allowing for the arrival and departure of armed U.S. air marshals. In accordance with its statutory authorities, however, FAMS may not deploy air marshals on foreign-flagged carriers.

[21] TSA designated further detail about these categories as sensitive security information and thus it cannot be included in a public report.

International: Flights covering international routes	International flights selected based on FAMS's assessment of the security risk of a flight's route or last point of departure.
National Special Security Events: Flights traveling into or out of cities during certain high- profile events	Flights associated with certain planned large gatherings that merit special security concern. These gatherings include events such as Presidential inaugurations and major international summits held in the United States. Transportation Security Administration is notified of these events and then identifies specific flights for FAMS coverage, depending on location, aircraft size, and other variables.
Random, Unpredictable: Flights not associated with other priority categories	Flights selected to maintain a periodic law enforcement presence on any type of domestic flight.
Special Mission Coverage: Flights for which a known, suspected, or potentially higher-risk traveler is ticketed	Flights selected based on specific intelligence about higher-risk or potentially higher-risk individual passengers, such as individuals who are in the federal government's database of known or suspected terrorists.
Supporting: Flights completed to support the coverage of other priority missions	Flights needed to position air marshals to cover a priority flight.

Source: GAO summary of FAMS operations documents I GAO-21-595.

To cover special mission coverage flights, FAMS typically uses air marshals scheduled for standby, who report to the airport or office and fly upon notification. If no air marshals in standby status are available, FAMS may reassign air marshals from regularly scheduled missions or air marshals who were not scheduled to fly at that time.

COVID-19 Effects on Flight and Passenger Volume

U.S. air carriers reduced both international and domestic flights in response to a decline in passenger demand following the onset of the pandemic, and TSA officials have publicly stated that they expect air travel to remain below pre-pandemic levels through most of 2021. In January 2020, the State Department and CDC began issuing a series of advisories to U.S. citizens discouraging certain domestic and international travel.[22] According to publicly available U.S. Department of Transportation flight data, in April 2020, U.S. air carriers decreased international flights to and from the U.S. by 93 percent and reduced domestic flights by 70 percent compared to pre-pandemic monthly averages.[23] U.S. air carrier flights have increased somewhat since April 2020, but as of November 2020—the most recent month for which Department of Transportation flight data were available at the time of our review—international flights to and from the U.S. remained at 34 percent of pre-pandemic levels and U.S. carrier domestic flights remained at 60 percent of pre-pandemic levels.[24] See figure 2.

FAMS Reported 345 Cases of COVID-19 through January 2021

FAMS reported 345 cases of COVID-19 among employees, including one death because of complications from COVID-19, as of January 31, 2021.[25] According to FAMS Medical Programs Section officials, this count captures all cases of COVID-19 confirmed by a positive diagnostic test.[26] FAMS has reported cases of COVID-19 in all 20 field offices and other FAMS work

---

[22] Specifically, in January 2020, the State Department advised U.S. citizens to avoid travel to China due to the novel coronavirus first identified in Wuhan, China. This travel advisory was extended in late February 2020 to include Italy due to evidence of community spread of the coronavirus. In March 2020, the CDC and State Department issued a Global Level 4 Health Advisory instructing U.S. citizens to avoid all international travel. From January through April 2020, the CDC issued recommendations for individuals to avoid discretionary domestic travel.

[23] For the purposes of this report, we define the "pre-pandemic" period as October 2019 through February 2020. Pre-pandemic flight levels are based on the number of average monthly passenger flights on U.S. carriers from October 2019 through February2020.

[24] The U.S. Department of Transportation reports publicly available passenger flight data on their website with a 3-month lag. Therefore, we analyzed passenger flight data through November 2020, the most recent month available at the time of our analysis.

[25] According to FAMS management officials, employees should communicate anypotential exposure to their immediate supervisor, but FAMS and TSA guidance do not require employees to do so. The TSA Human Capital Advisory Memo, and a March 12, 2020 email to the FAMS workforce, directed all employees to report any symptoms or possible exposure to COVID-19 to their local public health officials or healthcare provider.

[26] Each reported case generally represents a unique individual employee. Two employees had more than one case of COVID-19, representing four positive test results, as of January 2021.This case count includes all such cases reported to FAMS management, but may not include all cases that have occurred among employees. On July22, 2020, the CDC estimated that there were 10 times more cases than reported from March through May 2020.

locations, including their headquarters and training facilities. The infection rates per office ranged from less than 1 percent of employees in FAMS headquarters to 19 percent of employees in the Las Vegas field office. FAMS does not have information on how or where these employees caught COVID-19 and the TSA Chief Medical Officer said it would be nearly impossible to determine.[27] See figure 3 for the percent of employees in each field office who reported testing positive for COVID-19.

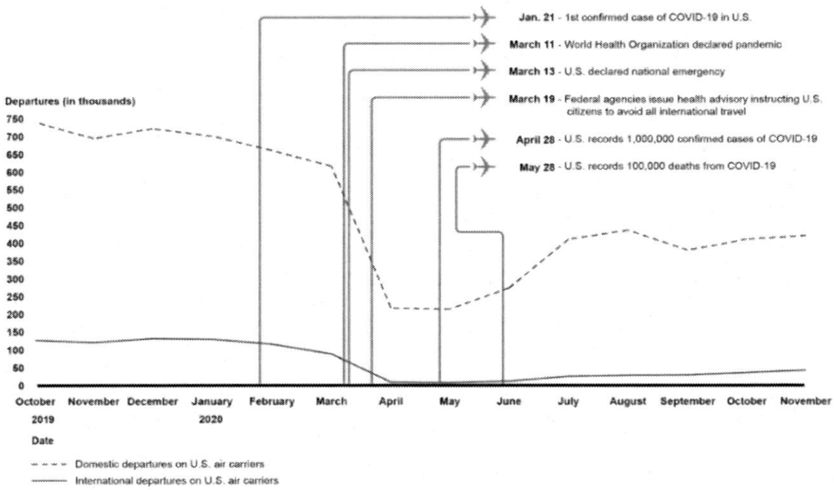

Source: GAO analysis of publicity available data from the Department of Transportation (departures); Centers for Desease Control and Prevention and John Hopkins University (COVID-19 cases and deaths). | GAO-21-595.

Figure 2. Numbers of Domestic and International Passenger Flights on U.S. Air Carriers, October 2019 – November 2020.

---

[27] The Department of Labor's Office of Workers' Compensation Programs has determined that for the purposes of the Federal Employees' Compensation Act, federal law enforcement officers—such as air marshals—whose employment causes them to come into direct and frequent in-person and close proximity contact with the public are assumed to have contacted COVID-19 as a result of their employment.

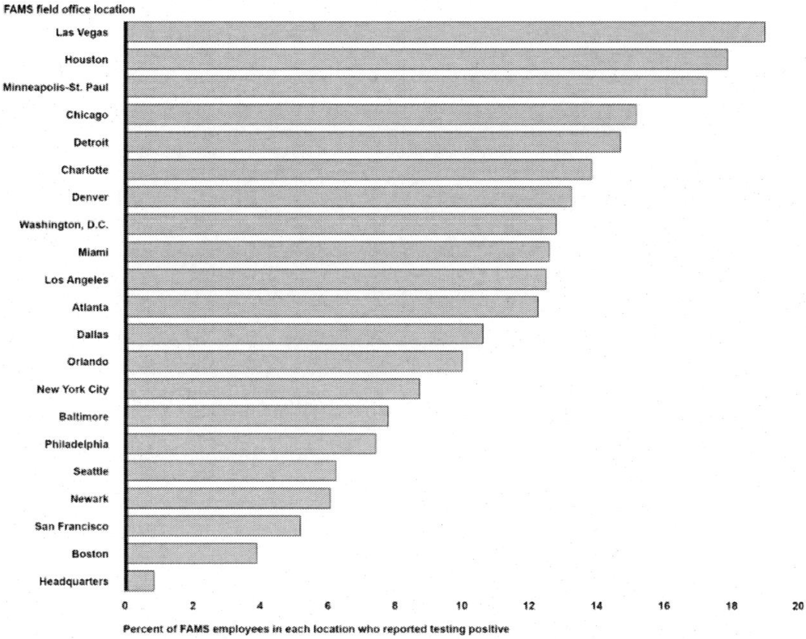

Source: GAO summary of FAMS COVID-19 case data. | GAO-21-595.

Note: Cases included here are reported confirmed cases of COVID-19 where an employee received a test and reported their positive test result to FAMS. This figure does not include 12 confirmed cases among FAMS employees located at the TSA Freedom Center in Herndon, Virginia and two reported cases of FAMS employees located at the Federal Law Enforcement Training Center in Artesia, New Mexico and the FAMS training facility in Atlantic City, New Jersey.

Figure 3. Percent of Federal Air Marshal Service (FAMS) Employees Who Reported Testing Positive for COVID-19 in Each Field Office, as of January 31, 2021.

According to our analysis of FAMS case data, the majority of COVID-19 infections occurred among flying air marshals (234 out of 345), while the remaining 111 cases occurred among employees in ground-based roles. Of these 111 cases, 50 occurred among field office supervisors and managers; 48 were among air marshals on ground-based assignments, such as VIPR; and 13 occurred among FAMS's administrative support staff.[28] Figure 4 shows the distribution of FAMS COVID-19 cases across different employee roles.

[28] These data reflect the job air marshals were doing when they reported their illness.

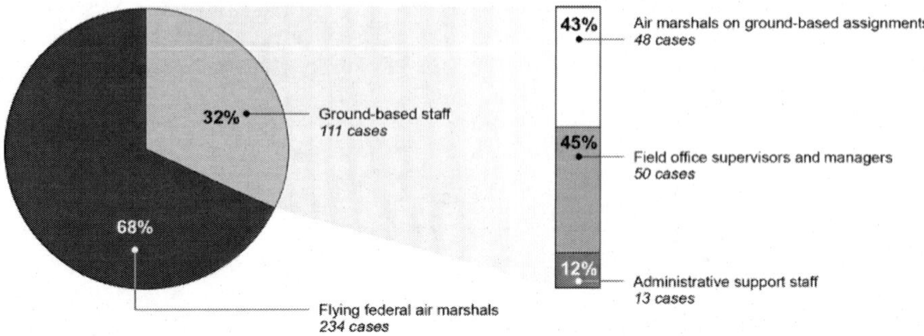

Source: GAO summary of FAMS COVID-19 case data. | GAO-21-595.

Note: Cases included here are reported confirmed cases of COVID-19 where an employee received a test and reported their positive test result to FAMS.

Figure 4. Distribution of Federal Air Marshal Service's (FAMS) Reported COVID-19 Cases by Employee Role, As of January 31, 2021.

FAMS Has Taken Steps to Protect Air Marshals, but Could Improve Documentation of These Efforts and Access to Testing

FAMS Has Taken Steps to Protect Employees during Travel and Ground-Based Work

FAMS has taken various steps to protect air marshals' health during the COVID-19 pandemic. Specifically, management has 1) provided Personal Protective Equipment (PPE), guidance, and adapted some travel procedures; 2) implemented new telework and leave policies; and 3) taken steps to reduce in-office contact.

FAMS Provided PPE, Guidance, and Adapted Some Travel Procedures

Beginning in January 2020, FAMS managers began to inventory, procure, and distribute PPE—including N95 masks, disinfectant wipes, and hand sanitizer—to air marshals, according to the Assistant Administrator for Field Operations. In February 2020, FAMS management emailed all air marshals notifying them that face coverings and other PPE were available for their use. Figure 5 shows PPE supplies available to air marshals in the Newark, New Jersey and Orlando, Florida field offices. By April 2020, the DHS Undersecretary for Management recommended all frontline workers—which includes FAMS—to wear a mask while on duty.[29] Starting in May 2020, the TSA Administrator required that all TSA employees— and specifically air marshals during flight operations—use masks during their work.

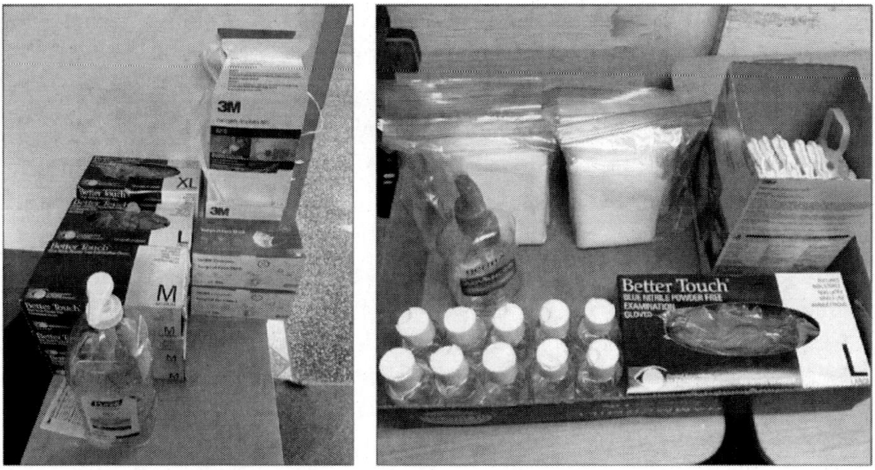

Source: Federal Air Marshal Service. | GAO-21-595.

Figure 5. Photos of N95 Masks, Hand Sanitizer, and Other Personal Protective Equipment Available to Federal Air Marshals.

Air marshals we met with in all three field offices said they had sufficient access to PPE. In one field office, the field office managers told us that in the midst of widespread shortages of travel-sized hand sanitizer, they emptied commercial-sized bottles of hand sanitizer into travel-sized bottles to ensure flying air marshals were able to get it. In another field office, the SAC told us they procured enough PPE locally to fulfill their needs and provide supplies to another field office. Air marshals in this field office told us that as of October 2020 they had various types of protective masks available for them to choose from, such as N95, surgical, and cloth reusable masks.

FAMS management officials also provided guidance to employees. In June 2020, the FAMS Safety Specialist—an official tasked with supporting air marshals' occupational safety and health—shared guidance with employees detailing safety precautions during travel. The guidance addressed, for example, steps to take to reduce COVID-19 risk when taking public transportation, staying at a hotel, and eating at restaurants. The guidance detailed basic hygiene principles and encouraged social distancing, among

[29] DHS provided this recommendation to all department employees by email on April 7, 2020.

other actions. The Safety Specialist also provided FAMS employees with links to CDC, World Health Organization, and other health groups' COVID-19 resources.

Individual field offices changed aspects of how air marshals work to encourage social distancing and reduce the risk of spreading COVID-19. For example, officials we spoke with in two of the three field offices told us to permit greater social distancing, SACs no longer required air marshals to be in the airport when assigned to standby, awaiting potential tasking to fly. Rather, these SACs allowed their air marshals to be outside of the airport, in their car, or at a nearby location.[30] According to air marshals and SACs in those two offices, this change improved air marshals' ability to socially distance without affecting the offices' abilities to complete their missions. In another example, the SAC of one field office we met with told us they had reduced the size of their VIPR teams, to decrease the number of coworkers exposed if one became infected with COVID-19 and to create more teams to ensure VIPR operations continued.

Beginning in January 2021, TSA and other federal agencies added to the steps already taken to protect air marshals. On January 5, 2021, TSA began offering COVID-19 vaccinations to mission critical frontline personnel, including the FAMS workforce, as part of the 1b vaccination priority group.[31] The vaccine distribution is part of a program with DHS and the Veterans Health Administration within the Department of Veterans Affairs. According to a TSA document, employees were to select whether they would receive the vaccine, but must notify their supervisors of their decision and whether they have already received the vaccine from another provider.[32] In addition, a January 21, 2021 Executive Order and subsequent Emergency Amendment by TSA, required that all individuals wear masks in airports, on planes, and in other transportation venues.[33]

---

[30] Air marshals staffed to "standby" roles were previously required to be in the airport to allow FAMS to fulfill missions with a different air marshal if unforeseen circumstances prevented the planned air marshal from travelling. In the remaining field office, the SAC did not implement this change, citing security priorities within the airport as the basis for continuing to require air marshals to be in the airport.

[31] According to CDC guidance, the allocation for COVID-19 vaccines designates phases for different groups. Specifically, the phase "1b" group includes individuals deemed frontline essential workers.

[32] We did not review FAMS's data on or monitoring of COVID-19 vaccination among the workforce. As of March 4, 2021, FAMS officials reported that 1,026 staff had received their first dose, and 681 of those had received both doses of the vaccine.

[33] White House. Executive Order on Promoting COVID-19 Safety in Domestic and International Travel. Exec. Order, 13998, 86 Fed. Reg. 7205 (Jan. 21, 2021). This Order also required a

FAMS Implemented New Telework and Leave Options

Prior to the pandemic, FAMS generally had not allowed air marshals to telework, but starting in March 2020, FAMS managers permitted and encouraged air marshals to telework when they did not need to be in the office.[34] On March 12, 2020, TSA issued its first *Human Capital Advisory Memo*, to guide the use of telework and various leave categories in response to COVID-19. This guidance encouraged employees—including FAMS employees—to use telework and other flexibilities to protect employees' health and well-being, protect the traveling public, and prevent the spread of COVID-19.

The March version of the TSA Human Capital Advisory Memo also provided that employees who had certain conditions (i.e., immunocompromised, asthma, etc.) and were therefore at a higher risk for negative outcomes from COVID-19 could use weather and safety leave.[35] In total, about 6 percent of the workforce took advantage of this option for some period of time. According to FAMS officials, FAMS did not schedule these individuals to fly or conduct in-person work while on weather and safety leave. An August 5, 2020 update to the TSA Human Capital Advisory Memo rescinded the use of weather and safety leave for high-risk employees.[36] TSA

---

negative COVID-19 test for passengers entering the country from international travel. On January 27, 2021, the Acting Secretary of DHS determined that a national emergency existed and directed TSA to take actions consistent with the authorities in Aviation and Transportation Security Act as codified at 49 U.S.C. sections 106(m) and 114(f), (g), (l), and (m) to implement the Executive Order to promote safety in and secure the transportation system. The mask order, which was due to expire May 11, 2021, was extended by TSA Emergency Amendment until September 13, 2021. TSA Emergency Amendment 1546-21-01A (April 30, 2021).

[34] TSA Management Directive 1100.30-5 Telework Program designated air marshals as emergency employees and therefore not eligible for routine telework. However, the Directive also states that under certain circumstances, employees occupying positions that are normally ineligible for telework may be considered for telework on a situational basis, limited to functions that are suitable for telework activity.

[35] According to TSA's human capital policies, prior to the pandemic, weather and safety leave was granted for employees when conditions—such as severe weather—made work or commuting unsafe.

[36] According to an email from the TSA Administrator to TSA employees, weather and safety leave was a tool to protect the highest-risk employees at the start of the pandemic; however, because of the increase in other protective measures, such as access to PPE, the risk of exposure had been reduced and TSA could revert to standard absence and leave policies. September 2020 updates to the Human Capital Advisory Memo (version 7) clarify procedures for the use of sick leave for employees who are at higher risk, at the suggestion of their doctor. December 2020 updates (version 8) further clarified the use of leave without pay for personal reasons, including health conditions that place the employee at higher risk. As of January 8, 2021, 10 air marshals continued to use a combination of sick leave, leave

clarified in a subsequent Human Capital Advisory Memo update that these employees could use sick leave at the suggestion of their doctor or leave without pay for personal reasons, including health reasons.

According to air marshals and SACs we met with in three field offices, the use of telework and other leave had helped protect air marshals' health and reduce the spread of COVID-19. For example, air marshals we met with in one office mentioned that they previously had to go to their office to complete time sheets and travel vouchers, but they were now able to do these tasks from home, thereby reducing their possible exposure to COVID-19.

FAMS Took Steps to Reduce In-Office Contact

FAMS also took steps intended to prevent the spread of COVID-19 in its offices and facilities, such as gyms and shooting ranges. In addition to reducing occupancy levels in the offices by promoting telework, FAMS closed all gyms and shooting range facilities in late March through July 2020. FAMS also waived training requirements for employees through June 2020.[37] On May 11, 2020, FAMS provided field offices with guidance for the reopening of its offices and gyms, based on the latest CDC and Occupational Safety and Health Administration guidelines. For example, FAMS recommended that field offices disinfect high-touch surfaces in their gyms every 2 hours, close showers and locker rooms, and follow masking and social distancing requirements, among other steps. Air marshals and managers in all three field offices we spoke with said their offices implemented these procedures, and others, such as sign-in procedures to control capacity limits in their facilities and other procedures to ensure social distancing.

FAMS Established Protocols for Responding to Cases, but Has Not Consistently Documented Implementation

In April 2020, TSA and FAMS management officials developed protocols to be followed when a FAMS employee reports a confirmed or suspected case of

---

without pay, or emergency paid sick leave, due to their risk for severe complications from COVID-19.

[37] Incumbent air marshals are required to complete 160 hours of recurrent training courses annually on such topics as use of force, defensive measures, firearms, mission tactics, and physical fitness. FAMS began reinstating training in August 2020, though employees were not required to attend training, according to a SAC we spoke to in one field office. According to the official, their office continued to delay training due to heightened COVID-19 levels in the community.

COVID-19.[38] The FAMS Protocols, a 3-page document, states, for example, that field office SACs must conduct contact tracing within the workforce; may contact airport officials in certain circumstances; and must contact local public health officials to report the case.[39] The TSA Chief Medical Officer and FAMS medical officer told us that they defer to local public health entities to handle or initiate any additional contact tracing.

The protocols also describe circumstances under which the field office SAC must notify other employees within the office that a coworker has tested positive for COVID-19.

The *FAMS Protocols* also instruct SACs to follow the TSA *Human Capital Advisory Memo* regarding the use of leave for quarantine when employees have been potentially exposed to COVID-19, and to follow TSA *Return to Workplace* guidance when determining the requirements for employees to return to work from a period of quarantine. This guidance explains TSA's criteria for an employee to return to work following different exposure situations. For example, an employee with a confirmed COVID-19 infection who remains asymptomatic may return to work after 10 days of quarantine from the employees' first positive test result.[40] Figure 6 describes the steps SACs and other FAMS employees are expected to take following a case of confirmed or suspected COVID-19 among their employees, as set forth in the *FAMS Protocols* and TSA guidance.

---

[38] FAMS defines a "suspected case" of COVID-19 to be cases where an employee (or contractor) has signs and symptoms clinically compatible with COVID-19, as identified by a healthcare provider, but the employee was not tested, or was tested and the test result is pending.

[39] According to FAMS management officials, there have been three revisions of the FAMS Protocols, first issued in April 2020. The FAMS Protocols does not provide information on the conditions under which SACs would have to contact airport officials. One SAC we spoke with described taking this step in a few cases, when the infected air marshals reported contact with someone at an airport. The FAMS Protocols also do not specify when SACs must carry out the steps but FAMS officials told us they expect contact tracing to be carried out as soon as practicable.

[40] None of the situations requires an employee to obtain a negative COVID-19 test result in order to return to work.

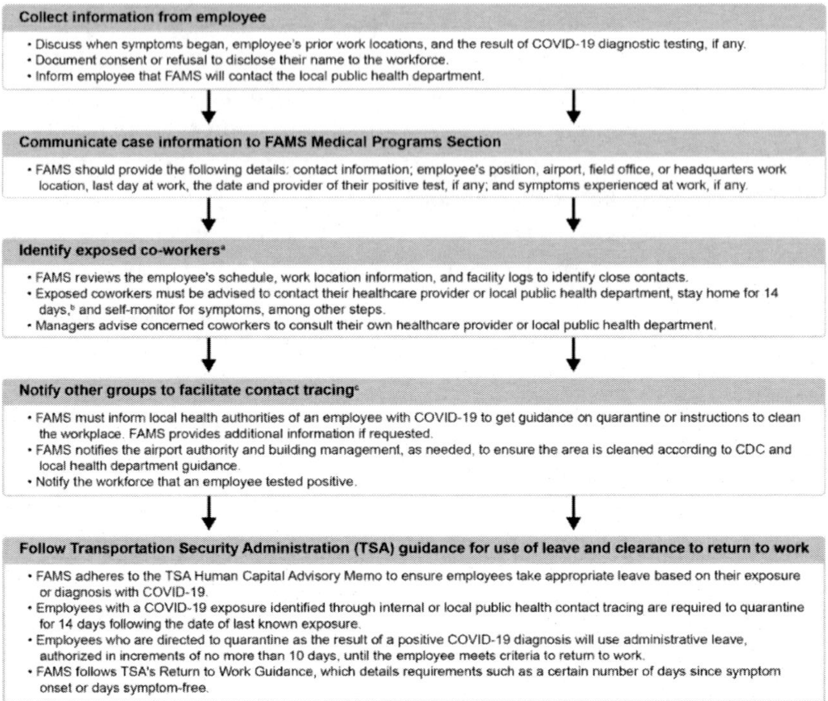

Source: GAO summary of FAMS and TSA guidance. | GAO-21-595.

[a]FAMS defines an "exposed coworker" as any employee who has had close contact with a symptomatic person or a person who has tested positive for COVID-19 without symptoms. FAMS defines "close contact" as within 6 feet for 15 minutes or more or being directly coughed on in the face.

[b]If exposed coworkers are mission-critical employees, FAMS leadership may assess whether they need to continue working, according to FAMS Protocols.

[c]FAMS defers to local public health entities to carry out any further contact tracing.

Figure 6. Federal Air Marshal Service (FAMS) Protocols for Responding to a COVID-19 Case.

FAMS has developed these protocols, but has not consistently documented their implementation. FAMS management provided us with examples of emails notifying field offices of COVID-19 cases—one of the steps in the protocols—but could not provide documentation showing implementation of other steps in the protocols. For example, they could not provide documentation of employees' consent or refusal to disclose their name to the workforce, a step that the FAMS protocols require be documented. Further, FAMS could not provide documentation confirming that required contact with local public health officials had been completed or that exposed coworkers had been advised to notify their healthcare providers. According to the Assistant Administrator for Field Operations, FAMS management has not seen a need to document the steps taken in response to cases of COVID-19. Rather, this official noted that they relied on verbal communication with field office SACs as a means to communicate about implementation of the protocols, as needed.

However, according to DHS *Risk Management Fundamentals*, leadership should require documentation of actions taken to implement a risk management strategy, specifically citing pandemics, such as COVID-19, as one source of risk. Further, according to *Standards for Internal Control in the Federal Government*, management should design control activities to achieve objectives and respond to risks. Internal control standards provide that one means of implementing this is for management to clearly document all transactions and other significant events in a manner that allows the documentation to be readily available for examination. Fully documenting the steps taken would facilitate FAMS management's oversight and better position them to assure both employees and the flying public that FAMS—a federal law enforcement entity tasked with protecting the public—is consistently taking the steps established in its protocols.

FAMS Does Not Routinely Facilitate Employee Access to Testing

FAMS recommends that employees who want or need COVID-19 testing seek it through their medical provider or local public health officials. Some air marshals told us they could be tested through their personal doctor or at local testing sites. However, air marshals in all three field offices we met with noted either barriers to testing or benefits to improved access to COVID-19 testing.[41] For example, air marshals we met with spoke of the time needed to wait in line in some communities and the length of time between being tested and obtaining results. These scheduling and timing challenges are particularly impactful for air marshals who may be scheduled to travel more than 50

[41] We reported in September 2020, that national challenges existed with testing supply availability and recommended the development of plans outlining specific actions the federal government could take to help mitigate remaining medical supply gaps—including testing supply shortages. See GAO, *COVID-19: Critical Vaccine Distribution, Supply Chain, Program Integrity, and Other Challenges Require Focused Federal Attention*, GAO-21-265 (Washington, D.C.: Jan. 28, 2021).

percent of their work days and may not be in a city—even their home city—for more than a few hours before their next flight.

Further, air marshals we met with expressed concern that they might be a threat to the public, because they are flying on multiple planes and through multiple cities every week, without knowing whether they might be asymptomatic and spreading COVID-19. A group of air marshals we spoke with in one office noted that this runs counter to their mission to protect the public. Lastly, representatives of all three employee groups we met with said that air marshals had persistent concerns about the lack of testing, which added to their stress given their fear of being at an increased risk of exposure or exposing family members to COVID-19.

Some FAMS employees and employee groups have shared resources to assist air marshals seeking COVID-19 testing. Air marshals we met with in one field office said that law enforcement workers, including air marshals, could access testing at a nearby location. According to them, an air marshal had identified this resource and shared it with their SAC; the SAC had then shared the information with others in the office. In another example, representatives from one employee group told us they were aware of a SAC in one field office who had compiled and shared a document with information about testing locations. FAMS management and Medical Programs Section officials told us they have in specific instances, such as when an employee is ill while on travel, helped an air marshal find a way to get tested, but said they do not routinely do this.

CDC guidance states that mitigation strategies such as social distancing and wearing masks continue to be important during the period of vaccination, and testing is one mitigation strategy that can help make travel safer, even though it does not eliminate all risk. Importantly, CDC guidance notes that even when individuals feel well and experience no symptoms, they may still spread COVID-19 to others in busy travel settings such as airports.[42] CDC guidance also states that experience from outbreaks in a variety of settings suggests that when symptomatic workers with COVID-19 are identified, there are often asymptomatic workers present in the workplace. According to the guidance, testing is important to identify such individuals, as they may not know they are infected and detecting workers earlier and excluding them from

[42] CDC "Domestic Travel during the COVID-19 Pandemic." December 2, 2020. Accessed December 14, 2020 at https://www.cdc.gov/coronavirus/2019-ncov/travelers/travel-during-covid19.html.

the workplace—that for air marshals includes airplanes and airports—can help prevent the spread of COVID-19.[43]

CDC guidance further states that testing before and after travel is a critical layer to slow the introduction and spread of COVID-19, particularly as variants of the virus continue to emerge in other countries. As such, in December 2020, the CDC recommended testing before and after domestic travel; and, effective January 26, 2021, began requiring all air passengers to provide a negative test result when they enter the country.[44] Guidance from the Occupational Safety and Health Administration also states that employers should provide information to workers about medical care, such as testing, in coordination with health insurance providers and local health agencies.[45]

FAMS management officials stated that they have not facilitated employee access to testing because they have not identified a need to do so. They noted that employees should be able to access COVID-19 testing through their private health providers or local health departments. One senior FAMS official noted that FAMS employees are not among the highest risk employees (like first responders) so they questioned whether limited testing resources should be used for air marshals and they further questioned the value of testing. However, one FAMS Medical Programs Section official stated that facilitated access to testing would be beneficial if it improves the timeliness of testing results for their employees. Further, according to DHS Human Capital officials, the Coast Guard and Secret Service are providing their employees with access to COVID-19 testing as part of their efforts to ensure

[43] CDC "Testing Strategies for Coronavirus (COVID-19) in High-Density Critical Infrastructure Workplaces after a COVID-19 Case is Identified, Testing in high-Density Critical Infrastructure Workplaces." June 13, 2020. Accessed October 14, 2020 at https://www.cdc.gov/coronavirus/2019-ncov/community/worker-safety-support/hd-testing.html.

[44] CDC guidance suggests getting a COVID-19 viral test 1 to 3 days prior to travel and within 3 to 5 days following a trip. Additionally, the CDC suggests reducing any non- essential activities for 7 to 10 days after traveling. See CDC "Domestic Travel during the COVID-19 Pandemic." December 2, 2020. Accessed December 12, 2020 at https://www.cdc.gov/coronavirus/2019-ncov/travelers/travel-during-covid19.html. CDC and Department of Health and Human Services. "Requirement for Negative Pre-Departure COVID-19 Test Result of Documentation of Recovery from COVID-19 For All Airline or Other Aircraft Passengers Arriving into the United Stated from Any Foreign Country". This order was issued pursuant to their authority under 42 C.F.R. § 71.20.

[45] Occupational Safety and Health Administration "Guidance on Preparing Workplaces for COVID-19." May 11, 2020. In additional guidance in January 2021, the Occupational Safety and Health Administration recommended that employers establish COVID-19 prevention programs and described 16 elements of effective programs, one of which is "providing guidance on screening and testing." See Occupational Safety and Health Administration. "Protecting Workers: Guidance on Mitigating and Preventing the Spread of COVID-19 in the Workplace". January 29, 2021.

continued operations during the pandemic, and DHS has provided all components with the opportunity to access a contract for COVID-19 testing as of January 2021. As of February 2021, FAMS did not plan to use this contract or otherwise facilitate employee access to testing. By routinely facilitating employee access to testing, FAMS would better support its workforce when employees want or need COVID-19 testing to ensure their health, the health of others, and continued operations during this exigent circumstance.

FAMS Adjusted Flight Coverage and Expanded Ground-Based Operations

Amidst Decline in U.S. Flight Volume, the Number of Flights FAMS Covered Declined 90 Percent in April 2020

In April 2020, amidst a 73 percent decline in total monthly domestic and international U.S. carrier flights,[46] the number of flights air marshals covered decreased by 90 percent compared to average monthly flights covered pre-pandemic.[47] With regard to international flights, specifically, in April 2020, when publicly available flight data indicate the total number of international flights on U.S. carriers had decreased 93 percent, air marshals covered no international flights.[48] This decline followed the first confirmed U.S. case of COVID-19 on January 21, 2020 and subsequent State Department and CDC travel advisories discouraging certain international travel starting in late January 2020.[49] (See figure 2) In response to these advisories, FAMS

[46] To determine trends in U.S. air carrier flight volume, we analyzed the U.S. Department of Transportation's publicly available passenger flight data.

[47] This decline in the number of flights FAMS covered is in part the result of the decrease in the total number of U.S. carrier international flights, and other high-priority domestic flights, as detailed below. For the purposes of this report, we define the "pre-pandemic" period as October 2019 through February 2020. TSA designated the specific numbers of flights FAMS covered as sensitive security information and thus they cannot be included in a public report.

[48] According to FAMS officials, many of the international flights they had planned to cover were cancelled during this period.

[49] Specifically, in January 2020, the State Department advised U.S. citizens to avoid travel to China due to the novel coronavirus first identified in Wuhan, China. This travel advisory was extended in late February 2020 to include Italy due to evidence of community spread of the coronavirus. In March 2020, the CDC and State Department issued a Global Level 4 Health Advisory instructing U.S. citizens to avoid all international travel.

management made a series of changes in the coverage of international missions through December 2020.[50]

- February 2020: FAMS management decided to stop covering certain international flights to China and Italy. In January 2020, the State Department advised U.S. citizens to avoid travel to China and in late February 2020, extended this advisory to include Italy.
- March and April 2020: According to FAMS officials, FAMS continued to deploy air marshals on international flights throughout the pandemic. However, because FAMS identified certain flights based on the risk associated with a specific passenger or passengers, the number of these international flights FAMS covered decreased as overall international passenger volume decreased in March and April 2020. Further, according to FAMS officials, in March 2020 they stopped coverage of certain international flights when the CDC and State Department issued a Global Level 4 Health Advisory instructing U.S. citizens to avoid all international travel. In effect, FAMS management did not have air marshals cover international flights for approximately 5 weeks.
- May 2020 through January 2021: From May 2020 through January 2021, as U.S. carrier flight volume increased, FAMS began covering certain international flights although at lower rates. FAMS officials reported that some of the international flights air marshals covered from May through January 2021 were in support of flights categorized as higher risk.

The number of domestic flights air marshals covered in April 2020 was 88 percent lower than average monthly domestic flights covered pre-pandemic. According to FAMS officials and our analysis of publicly available flight data, this decrease reflects both the 70 percent reduction in U.S. carriers' total domestic flights and the specific reductions in flights FAMS categorizes as National Special Security Events and Special Mission Coverage. With regard to National Special Security Events, CDC guidance on limiting the size of events and public concern about the pandemic caused many of these events to be cancelled or conducted in virtual environments. As a result, FAMS conducted no flights related to National Special Security Events from March

[50] TSA designated the details of FAMS's changes to flight operations as sensitive security information and thus they cannot be included in a public report.

through June 2020. With regard to Special Mission Coverage, with fewer passengers flying, FAMS saw a corresponding decrease in flights with higher risk travelers.

FAMS Adjusted the Types of Flights It Covered and Increased Ground-Based Activities

FAMS Increased Flights to Pre-Pandemic Levels by June 2020

Beginning in April 2020, FAMS management implemented operational changes to increase the number of monthly covered flights.[51] They did this in part, by increasing the number of flights they covered that do not fit FAMS's defined flight categories. For example, FAMS data indicate that air marshals covered more random, unpredictable flights in June 2020 than pre-pandemic.[52] Following these operational changes, by June 2020, FAMS covered approximately the same number of flights per month as it did on average in pre-pandemic months; however, the types of flights covered differed.[53]

FAMS Has Continued to Adapt Flight Operations

From July 2020 through January 2021, the number and types of flights FAMS covered continued to fluctuate in response to ongoing changes in the airline industry and FAMS management's decisions to end some flight operations modifications, among other variables.

From July 2020 through January 2021, the number of flights FAMS covered per month varied from a high in August 2020 to a low in December 2020. FAMS officials explained that the high number of flights covered in August was the result of the increase in total U.S. domestic flights combined with their April and May 2020 decisions to expand the types of flights FAMS would cover. They explained that due to instability in the airline industry, it had been difficult for FAMS leadership to predict how the changes in their flight selection criteria would affect the total number of covered flights.

---

[51] TSA designated the details of FAMS's operational changes as sensitive security information and thus they cannot be included in a public report.

[52] Prior to the pandemic, in addition to their defined flight categories, FAMS scheduled random, unpredictable flights based on air marshals' availability. According to FAMS officials, in March 2020, in response to the pandemic, they discontinued these flights. Starting in May 2020, FAMS categorized all flights that did not meet the conventional definitions of their flight categories as random, unpredictable flights.

[53] TSA designated the specific number of flights air marshals covered as sensitive security information and thus it cannot be included in a public report.

According to FAMS officials and documentation, in August 2020, FAMS leadership adopted two changes they expected would reduce the number of covered flights going forward.

FAMS covered fewer flights in December 2020 in part because of increased COVID-19 infection rates in certain cities, according to FAMS management officials. Beginning in July 2020, FAMS tracked the level of COVID-19 infection by city and restricted operations that would require air marshals to stay overnight in locations with high rates of infection—which they referred to as "hotspots."[54] According to FAMS officials, FAMS's coverage of flights in January 2021 increased, in part, due to additional flight coverage following the January 6, 2021 attack on the U.S. Capitol and increased coverage associated with the January 20, 2021 Presidential Inauguration, a National Special Security Event.[55]

As of February 2021, FAMS officials reported that they were not covering certain international flights due to CDC travel advisories, but were otherwise selecting flights for coverage much as they had pre- pandemic.[56] FAMS officials explained that they did not anticipate FAMS would be covering flights at pre-pandemic levels given the decrease in U.S. air travel, but they were not working toward a specific target number of covered flights per month. As of February 2021, FAMS officials told us they were not planning any modifications to their flight operations.

FAMS Plans to Permanently Increase Ground-Based Activities

FAMS leadership is in the early stages of planning to permanently shift operations toward more ground-based transportation security activities. According to the Executive Assistant Administrator/Director of FAMS, FAMS leadership had been considering an increase in ground-based operations prior to the COVID-19 pandemic—as far back as 2011—but the effects of the COVID-19 pandemic have caused them to accelerate this shift.

---

[54] According to FAMS officials and documentation, beginning in July 2020, FAMS worked with TSA's Intelligence and Analysis Office, and assessed data from the Johns Hopkins Coronavirus Resource Center to determine the weekly level of COVID-19 infection in the areas around U.S. airports. FAMS officials explained that FAMS generally discontinued overnight stays in these areas but in certain circumstances, such as a lengthy operation or in the event of weather delays, air marshals were asked to stay overnight in a hotel near the airport.

[55] According to FAMS officials, air marshals covered hundreds of flights in January 2021 related to the heightened security following the January 6, 2021 attack on the U.S. Capitol and the Presidential Inauguration. TSA designated the specific number of flights as sensitive security information and thus it cannot be included in a public report.

[56] FAMS continued to track hotspot airports and avoid overnight missions in those areas.

In April 2020, when FAMS flight operations were at decreased levels, FAMS leadership increased air marshals' participation in some ground- based activities such as expanded VIPR operations and supporting TSA and DHS activities.

- *Expanding VIPR work.* According to FAMS officials, FAMS expanded VIPR operations in at least four field offices by deploying at least 47 air marshals to enhance transportation security and free up local law enforcement for other purposes.[57] For example, leadership of the Seattle field office told us that during a period when they had fewer air marshals on flights, they deployed air marshals to aid with VIPR operations at transportation venues when the Seattle Police Department was focused on local civil unrest.
- *Supporting TSA at airports.* Prior to the pandemic, FAMS regularly supported TSA at airports with duties including overt and covert law enforcement activities. According to FAMS officials, in April 2020 air marshals increased their support for TSA operations in some airports. For example, from April through July 2020, in Newark, New Jersey, air marshals worked additional shifts at the airport to provide exit lane security when there was a shortage of Transportation Security Officers due to COVID-19. FAMS officials told us that at least 134 air marshals across ten field offices have provided support to TSA at airports since April 2020. FAMS officials told us that they also increased their security assistance at small-hub airports.[58] According to FAMS management officials, prior to COVID-19, FAMS did not typically assist TSA in this manner. However, starting in April 2020 FAMS officials said that they regularly deployed eight air marshals to these two airports to provide security assistance.[59] FAMS also deployed four air marshals from the Boston,

[57] FAMS management officials explained that they provided field office management with discretion in how they utilized VIPR operations during this time, so they did not have comprehensive data on the extent of FAMS's VIPR operations agency-wide. Rather, FAMS officials asked field office management retrospectively about their VIPR operations during this period and identified that at least 47 air marshals in four offices were assigned to support VIPR operations from inception of the pandemic through October 2020.

[58] Federal law defines a small-hub airport as an airport with scheduled air carrier service that receives 0.05 to 0.25 percent of the annual U.S. commercial enplanements.49 U.S.C.§ 40102(a)(42).

[59] As of January 2021, FAMS officials stated that one air marshal based out of the Washington field office was providing ongoing to support to TSA at the Norfolk, Virginia airport and FAMS was providing support to TSA at the Richmond, Virginia airport upon request.

Massachusetts field office to three regional airports from May through December 2020 and five air marshals from the New York City, New York field office to three regional airports from June through August 2020 to provide on- going security assistance.

- *Supporting other DHS activities.* FAMS officials told us that at least 339 air marshals provided support to other DHS components from April through December 2020. For example, FAMS officials told us that in March 2020, they deployed VIPR teams of air marshals from six field offices to support Federal Emergency Management Agency by providing security and safe escort for individuals quarantined at Joint Base Lackland and Travis Air Force Base.[60] FAMS also deployed 18 air marshals to assist the Federal Protective Service with responsibilities such as protecting federal property at Gettysburg National Battleground on July 4, 2020. Additionally, FAMS officials told us that from August through December 2020, approximately, 285 air marshals supported the U.S. Secret Service in a variety of assignments including providing security at the Democratic National Convention.

In January 2021, FAMS further expanded its ground-based activities. Specifically, FAMS officials told us that following the January 6, 2021 attack on the U.S. Capitol, VIPR teams from the Washington and Baltimore field offices supported TSA by providing an increased visible law enforcement presence at airport screening checkpoints and provided protective escorts for congressional members, staff, and others (see figure 10). Further, for the January 20, 2021 Presidential Inauguration, eight FAMS VIPR teams supported DHS Countering Weapons of Mass Destruction Mobile Detection Deployment Units and 224 air marshals supported the U.S. Secret Service through assignments including providing security at inauguration venues.[61]

---

[60] FAMS deployed VIPR teams from Chicago, Illinois; Los Angeles, California; New York City, New York; San Francisco, California; Seattle, Washington; and Washington, D.C. to assist with quarantine efforts from March 10-26, 2020.

[61] Within DHS, the Domestic Nuclear Detection Office deploys Mobile Detection Deployment Units—radiological and nuclear detection equipment housed in a mobile trailer package—as a national surge asset, designed to augment and supplement first responders' existing capabilities, especially in support of national and special security events. According to FAMS officials, the eight VIPR teams conducted 42 operations from January 17-22, 2021 in support of Amtrak, Maryland Area Regional Commuter, Washington Metropolitan Area Transit Authority, and the Metropolitan Washington Airport Authority.

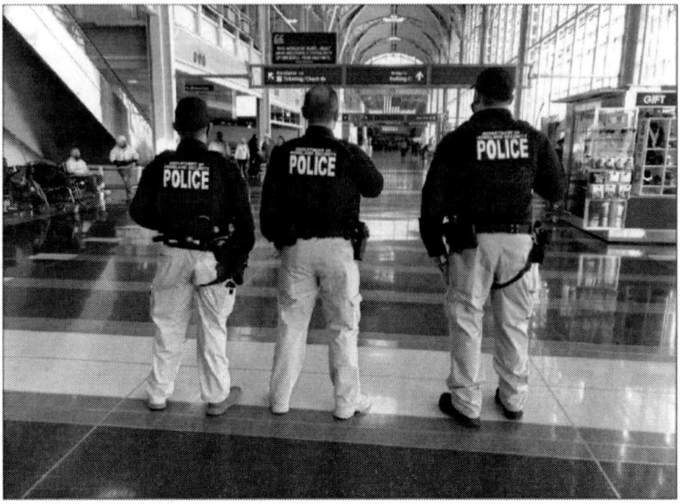

Source: Transportation Security Agency. | GAO—21-595.

Figure 7. Federal Air Marshals Support Inauguration Event Security at Ronald Reagan Washington National Airport.

The FAMS Director said the purpose of this shift toward more ground-based activities is to find additional ways for air marshals to contribute to DHS and TSA security missions in a changing national security environment. FAMS leadership also intends for the shift toward a greater variety of law enforcement tasks to benefit employee retention and morale.

FAMS leadership has tasked a working group with identifying opportunities for air marshals to engage in new ground-based initiatives, such as participating in TSA red-team testing, assisting with behavior detection activities at airport security checkpoints, working with airport officials on access control, and assisting with passenger screening at airport departure gates.[62] The FAMS Director said he anticipated FAMS would not need any additional authorities to carry out these changes. In November 2020, the working group reported 12 recommendations for FAMS leadership and, as of

[62] What TSA commonly calls "red team" tests are covert tests that are designed to assess TSA's screening operations. Behavior detection is a technique used by TSA to identify passengers exhibiting behaviors indicative of stress, fear, or deception at airport screening checkpoints. According to TSA, certain verbal and nonverbal cues and behaviors may indicate mal-intent and provide a means for identifying passengers who may pose a risk to aviation security and referring them for additional screening. GAO has issued numerous reports about TSA's use of behavior detection, most recently GAO, *Aviation Security: TSA Has Policies that Prohibit Unlawful Profiling But Should Improve Its Oversight of Behavior Detection Activities,* GAO-19-268 (Washington, D.C.: Apr. 23, 2019).

January 2021, FAMS leadership had named a program manager to lead the development and implementation of the operational changes. FAMS officials said they expected to begin implementing the changes on a rolling basis through 2021 and they planned to update their concept of operations to reflect the changes.

Conclusion

The COVID-19 pandemic has resulted in catastrophic loss of life. Public health officials have widely recommended physical distancing to reduce transmission, but air marshals' jobs require that they work at airports, on airplanes, and in other public spaces where they are routinely in close quarters with colleagues and the public. To mitigate this risk, FAMS has taken steps intended to help protect employees from infection at work, such as providing PPE and encouraging employees to telework. Even with these and other measures, FAMS reports that, as of January 31, 2021, 345 employees had been infected with COVID-19 and one air marshal had died due to complications of the disease.

FAMS developed and implemented protocols to guide its response when employees became sick with COVID-19, but has not consistently documented the steps taken to implement the protocols. Doing so would facilitate management oversight and better position FAMS to assure both its employees and the flying public that it is consistently implementing its protocols.

FAMS recommends that employees seek COVID-19 testing through their medical provider or local public health officials but air marshals we met with noted barriers to testing and benefits to improved access. In January 2021, FAMS employees became eligible for COVID-19 vaccinations through the Department of Veterans Affairs, but CDC guidance says testing continues to be important even as vaccinations become available. By facilitating employee access to testing, FAMS would better support its workforce to ensure their health, the health of others, and continued operations during this exigent circumstance.

Recommendations for Executive Action

We are making the following two recommendations to FAMS:

- The Executive Assistant Administrator/Director of FAMS should ensure that FAMS officials consistently document steps taken to implement agency protocols following identification of employees with COVID-19. (Recommendation 1).
- The Executive Assistant Administrator/Director of FAMS should routinely facilitate employee access to COVID-19 testing. (Recommendation 2).

Agency Comments and Our Evaluation

We provided a draft of our report to DHS for comment. In written comments, which are included in Appendix I, the agency concurred with our two recommendations and described steps they plan to take to address them. DHS also provided technical comments, which we have incorporated, as appropriate.

With regard to our first recommendation that FAMS consistently document steps taken to implement agency protocols following identification of employees with COVID-19, DHS responded that it would develop and implement a formal reporting process to document the steps taken at FAMS field offices and headquarters by the end of June 2021. If implemented effectively, this would address the intent of our recommendation.

With regard to our second recommendation that FAMS routinely facilitate employee access to COVID-19 testing, DHS responded that it would provide information to employees regarding available COVID-19 testing locations, and ensure that employees deployed away from home have the necessary assistance to obtain testing by the end of June 2021. If implemented effectively, this would address the intent of our recommendation.

We are sending copies of this report to the appropriate congressional committees, the Secretary of Homeland Security, and other interested parties.

In addition, the report is available at no charge on the GAO website at http://www.gao.gov.

If you or your staff have any questions about this report, please contact me at (202) 512-8777 or McNeilT@gao.gov. Contact points for our Office of Congressional Relations and Public Affairs may be found on the last page of this report. Key contributors to this report are listed in appendix IV.

Triana McNeil

Director, Homeland Security and Justice

List of Committees

The Honorable Patrick Leahy
Chairman

The Honorable Richard Shelby
Vice Chairman
Committee on Appropriations,
United States Senate

The Honorable Ron Wyden
Chairman

The Honorable Mike Crapo
Ranking Member
Committee on Finance United
States Senate

The Honorable Patty Murray
Chair

The Honorable Richard Burr
Ranking Member
Committee on Health, Education,
Labor, and Pensions
United States Senate
The Honorable Gary C. Peters
Chair

The Honorable Rob Portman
Ranking Member
Committee on Homeland Security
and Governmental Affairs,
United States Senate

The Honorable Rosa L. DeLauro
Chairwoman

The Honorable Kay Granger
Ranking Member
Committee on Appropriations,
House of Representatives

The Honorable Frank Pallone, Jr.
Chairman

The Honorable Cathy McMorris
Rodgers
Republican Leader
Committee on Energy and
Commerce, House of
Representatives

The Honorable Bennie G.
Thompson
Chairman

The Honorable John Katko
Ranking Member
Committee on Homeland Security,
House of Representatives

The Honorable Carolyn B. Maloney
Chairwoman
The Honorable James Comer
Ranking Member
Committee on Oversight and
Reform, House of Representatives

The Honorable Richard Neal
Chair

The Honorable Kevin Brady
Republican Leader
Committee on Ways and Means,
House of Representatives

Appendix I: Comments from the Department of Homeland Security

U.S. Department of Homeland Security
Washington, DC 20528

Homeland Security

June 4, 2021

Triana McNeil
Director, Homeland Security and Justice
U.S. Government Accountability Office
441 G Street, NW
Washington, DC 20548

Re: Management Response to Draft Report GAO-21-595, "COVID-19: Federal Air Marshal Service Should Document Its Response to Cases and Facilitate Access to Testing"

Dear Ms. McNeil:

Thank you for the opportunity to comment on this draft report. The U.S. Department of Homeland Security (DHS or the Department) appreciates the U.S. Government Accountability Office's (GAO) work in planning and conducting its review and issuing this report.

The Department is pleased to note GAO's positive recognition of the actions taken by the Transportation Security Administration's (TSA) Federal Air Marshal Service (FAMS) to mitigate the impacts of COVID-19 to help keep its workforce safe and to maintain transportation security throughout the Nation, such as providing employees personal protective equipment and encouraging them to telework. While the pandemic persists, TSA's mitigation efforts continue to improve as preventative resources, such as the availability of vaccinations, become more readily available. Likewise, lessons learned involving employee safety protocols and medical reporting have helped improve DHS processes for dealing with wide-spread health pandemics.

The draft report contained two recommendations with which the Department concurs. Attached find our detailed response to each recommendation. DHS previously submitted technical comments addressing several accuracy, contextual, and other issues under a separate cover for GAO's consideration.

Again, thank you for the opportunity to review and comment on this draft report. Please feel free to contact me if you have any questions. We look forward to working with you again in the future.

Sincerely,

JIM H CRUMPACKER Digitally signed by JIM H CRUMPACKER Date: 2021.06.04 10:44:35 -04'00'

JIM H. CRUMPACKER, CIA, CFE
Director
Departmental GAO-OIG Liaison Office

Attachment

Attachment: Management Response to Recommendations Contained in GAO-21-595

GAO recommended that the Executive Assistant Administrator/Director of FAMS:

Recommendation 1: Ensure that FAMS officials consistently document steps taken to implement agency protocols following identification of employees with COVID-19.

Response: Concur. TSA's FAMS will develop and implement a formal reporting process documenting: (1) agency protocols taken at each field office location and other FAMS facilities, including headquarters offices; and (2) positive COVID-19 diagnoses of employees. Estimated Completion Date (ECD): June 30, 2021.

Recommendation 2: Routinely facilitate employee access to COVID-19 testing.

Response: Concur. TSA's FAMS will provide information to employees regarding available COVID-19 testing locations, and will also ensure that employees deployed away from their homes have the necessary assistance to obtain testing. ECD: June 30, 2021

3

Appendix II: Staff Acknowledgments

In addition to the contact named above, Claudia Becker (Assistant Director), Amanda Parker (Analyst in Charge), Paul Aussendorf, Karen Doran, Clifton Douglas, Elizabeth Dretsch, David Hooper, Susan Irving, Tyler Kent, Terell Lasane, Diona Martyn, Adam Vogt, and Emilie Weisser made key contributions to this report.

Index

D

E

F

G

H

Q

R

S

W